working with chi

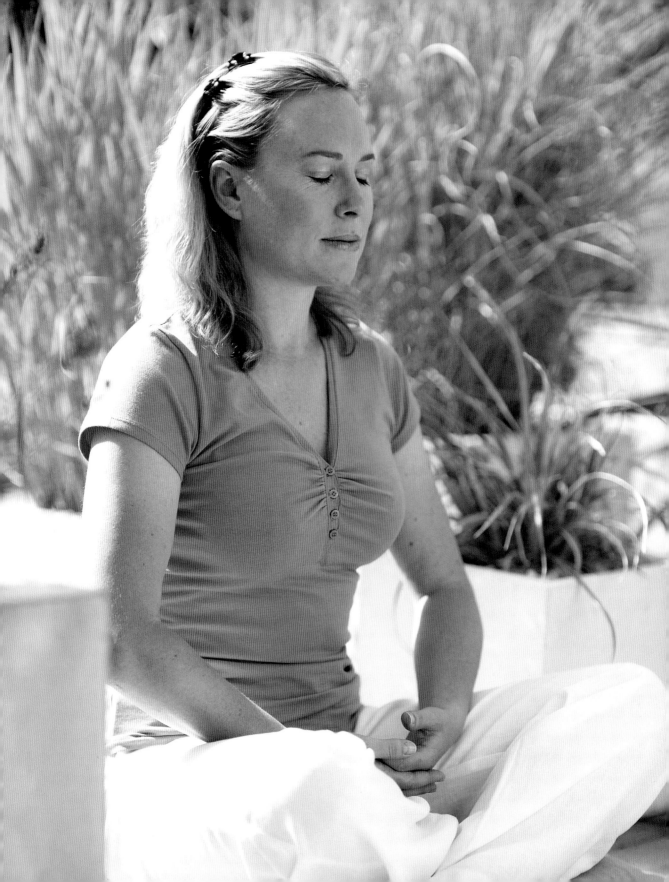

working with chi

practical ways to harness healing energy

Madonna Gauding

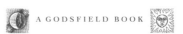

A GODSFIELD BOOK

An Hachette Livre UK Company
www.hachettelivre.co.uk

First published in Great Britain
in 2008 by Godsfield Press, a division
of Octopus Publishing Group Ltd
2–4 Heron Quays,
London E14 4JP
www.octopusbooks.co.uk

Distributed in the United States and
Canada by Hachette Book Group
USA, 237 Park Avenue, New York, NY
10017 USA

ISBN: 978-1-84181-332-5

A CIP catalogue record for this book
is available from the British Library.

Printed and bound in China

10 9 8 7 6 5 4 3 2 1

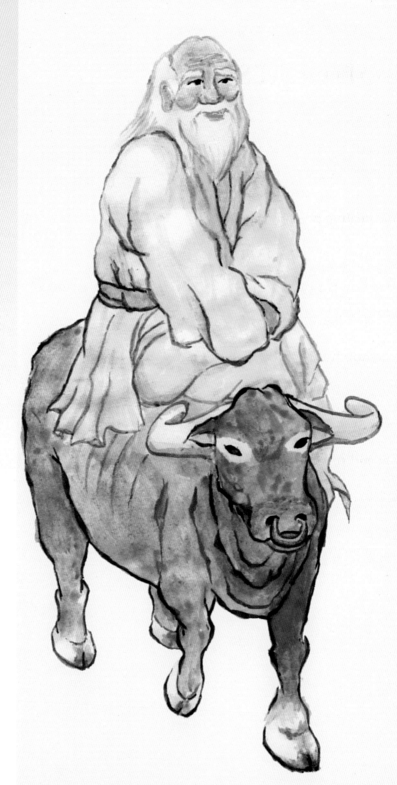

contents

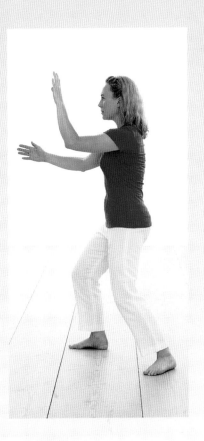

INTRODUCTION

The word 'chi' means 'breath'. According to ancient Eastern thought, chi is the breath of life that animates everything on this planet. It is the essence or soul of all things, and the energy that causes activity and change throughout the universe, not only in animate living things but also in the inanimate world that surrounds us. This book aims to whet your appetite for learning more about an ancient form of energy. It will teach you how to begin to work with chi to enhance your health and well-being using diet, exercise and meditative practices.

A simple, clear explanation of chi and its place in Chinese Taoist culture is provided in the first chapter. How chi works with yin and yang, a look at Chinese Taoist philosophy and the Three Treasures of the human being are also covered and will add to an understanding of chi and its role within your life.

The fluids you drink and the foods you eat affect the flow of chi throughout your body.

Chinese medicine

A traditional Chinese doctor adopts an energetic view of the body and uses the eight principles of Chinese medicine to diagnose illness. Chapter 2 shows how you can assess the state of your own chi by understanding the three sources, the four kinds and the three states of chi. An introduction to the Chinese Five Element System, and how each of the elements manifests in the body in states of harmony or illness is discussed in the third chapter and you can learn how to determine your dominant element.

The flow of chi throughout the body is facilitated by major chi pathways or meridians, each of which governs an organ system and is related to the five elements. The flow of chi can be balanced through massage of the meridians to restore health and instructions on how to do this are given in chapter 4. Diet also plays a key role in health – the chi in food and the concept of yin and yang as it relates to diet are also examined. Learning how chi, the five elements and the meridians are linked to proper nutrition can help you to determine the best diet for your own needs.

relaxation, exercise and a spiritual path

The flow of chi can be altered and improved through relaxation and exercise. The chi energy practices of Chi Kung and T'ai Chi, with accompanying exercises that are given in chapter 8, allow you to balance chi through physical movement, while the chi meditation practices in the final chapter let you explore your own path to spiritual enlightenment.

This simple yet profoundly powerful force that shapes everything in the universe is worthy of a lifetime's study, but this book will introduce you to its basic ideas and teach you to use its concepts to enhance your life.

Chi Kung and T'ai Chi exercises are excellent energy practices for enhancing and balancing the flow of chi.

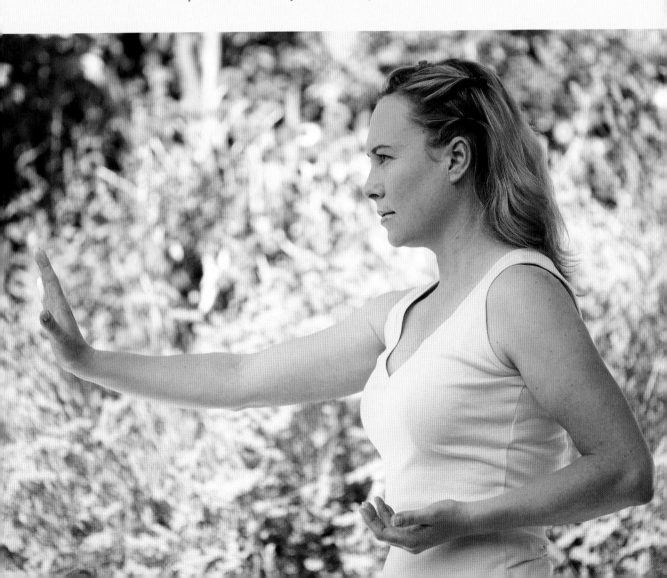

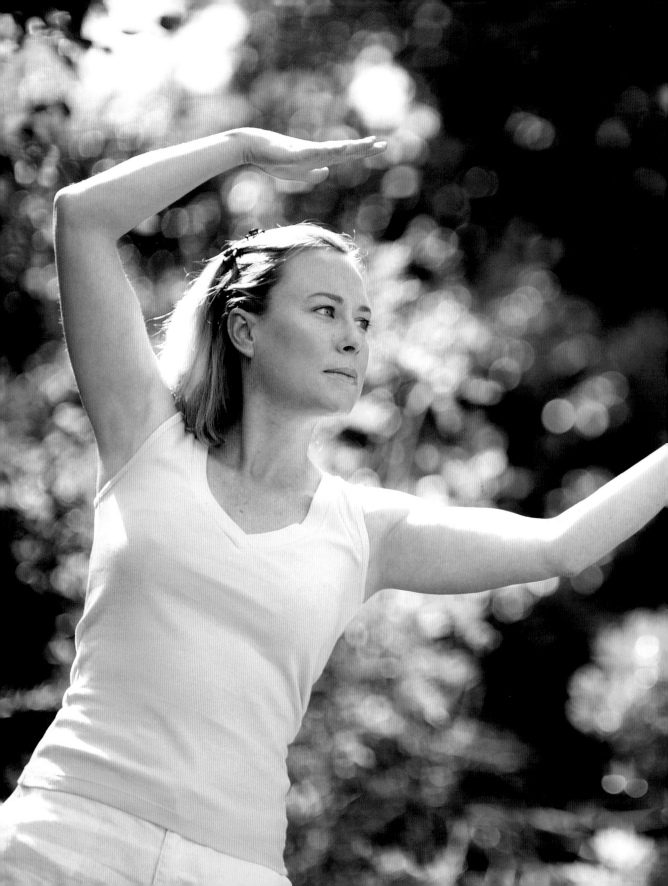

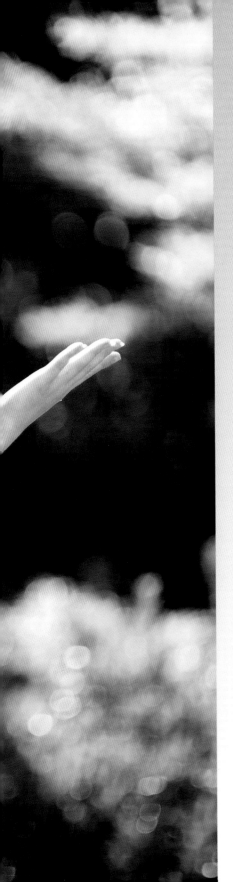

WHAT IS CHI?

The Chinese word chi means breath or vapour – in fact, the Chinese character for chi depicts steam rising from a pot of cooked rice. The word and character are unremarkable, yet what they symbolize and describe is breathtakingly profound. Chi is the energy that animates all life and the unifying substance or soul of all things. It is sometimes called 'life's breath', and is the force that causes all activity and change in the universe in both animate and inanimate things. It is the very life-energy that flows through your body and it inhabits all matter and space around you. Chi is so essential to life that without it you cease to exist.

the concept of chi

The concept of chi is very ancient and dates back thousands of years in Chinese history. The *I Ching* or *Book of Changes*, an ancient text with many authors and evolved over thousands of years, contains the first references to chi where it is described as an all-encompassing force that pervades and unifies the three energies in the universe – heaven, earth and human. The first known date for the *Book of Changes* is about 2200 BCE. Under King Wen (c.1150 BCE), the founder of the Chou Dynasty, the present form of the *I Ching* was written.

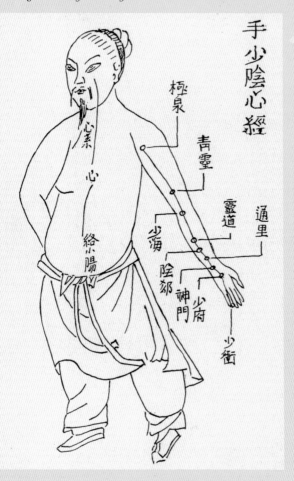

An ancient Chinese drawing showing the points along the heart meridian, the pathway of chi that governs the function of the heart.

beyond measurement

Chi is difficult to measure in Western terms because it can't be quantified in any way. It can't be seen with the naked eye or captured on an x-ray or in a test tube. Because it is difficult to define, it is often described by what it causes and affects rather than what it is. The chi of the sun allowing life on earth; the chi of changing weather patterns producing moisture and allowing crops to grow; and chi flowing through the meridians in the body, supporting life, preventing disease and enhancing wellness are all examples of chi's effects.

Chi is an energy that manifests as sound, light, emotion, thought, mountains, trees, rivers, weather, digestion, movement and heat. It is often compared to the wind in the sail; we do not see the wind directly but we see its effect as it fills the sail of a boat.

invisible forces

These descriptions may sound mysterious, Eastern and mystical. But the concept of invisible energies is not unique to the East. Western scientists have identified invisible forces such as electricity, x-rays, radioactivity

may the force be with you

The idea of a life-energy or a life-force inherent in all living things is not exclusive to China. It is a concept and archetype expressed in many cultures around the world; even George Lucas, in his modern-day science-fiction films *Star Wars*, had a name for it – he called it 'the force'. Below are the names given to chi in various countries and cultures:

- Japan – ki
- India – prana
- Polynesia – mana
- Egyptian mythology – ka
- Greek mythology and in Christianity – pneuma
- African Yoruba mythology – ashe.

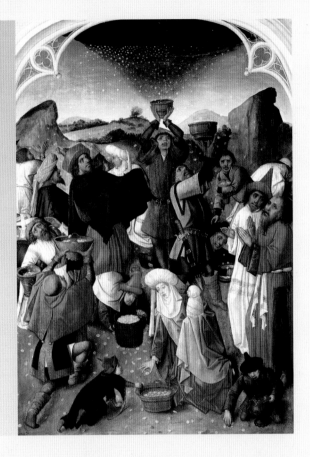

The idea of an invisible energy force is found in the Western European tradition.

and subatomic particles. In the Eastern view, these invisible energies are all manifestations of chi. While modern scientists have not yet proven the existence of chi in the body, they have confirmed that the acupoints, the gateways of chi along the meridians, have a stronger electrical potential than the surrounding tissue. Both Eastern and Western researchers are optimistic that someday they will prove scientifically the existence of chi energy and its meridian pathways in the body, which have been accepted as fact in Asian cultures for thousands of years.

All cultures have some concept of a life-force, but it is in China where we find the most sophisticated understanding of this invisible energy. From the Chinese we can learn how to work with chi to maintain and improve our physical, mental and spiritual health and well-being. As you will discover, learning to manage chi through diet, exercise and meditation is one of the most important life skills you can acquire.

where does chi come from?

The Chinese consider chi to be a kind of primordial energy that has always existed and will always exist. According to ancient Chinese Taoist philosophy, before our universe came into being, there was 'Wu Chi' or a kind of pregnant void from which all things become possible. That pregnant void contained the potential for the creation or manifestation of all things, and embodied all the physical laws necessary for any kind of universe that might emerge.

From that void, or state of Wu Chi, our universe was born as a consequence of the 'Great Separation' – the emergence of the positive and negative forces of yin and yang. These two forces were then driven by the ever-present chi in a continuing and never-ending dance of creation, transformation and balance.

chi and quantum physics

The idea of chi is similar to the Western concept of the quantum field in modern physics. Like the quantum field, chi manifests simultaneously as energy and matter, particle and wave, and is the underlying essence of all living and non-living things. On the origin of the universe, however, Western science has a different view. The Big Bang theory holds that the universe is expanding but will eventually collapse in on itself and end. The Chinese have a more positive and perhaps gentler view. According to Taoist thought, if the universe as we know it ends, it will simply revert to another state of Wu Chi, or pregnant void, out of which another universe or universes will emerge.

feeling chi energy

1 An easy and simple way to begin to feel chi energy flow in your body is to stand up and stretch. Do it now. Notice how energizing it is to stretch. This is because gentle stretching opens the pathways or meridians in your body through which flow chi energy.

2 Now breathe deeply into your lower abdomen. Deep breathing leads to relaxation, which encourages the smooth flow of chi in your body.

3 Hold your arms straight out in front of you with palms facing each other a few centimetres or inches apart. As you breathe in move your palms apart, and when you breathe out move them back to the original position, without touching. Do this several times and you should begin to feel chi energy as heat radiating between your palms.

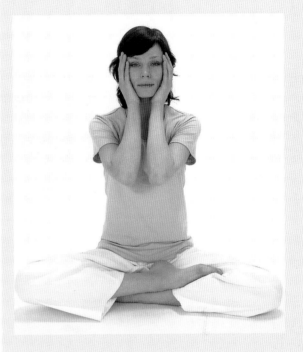

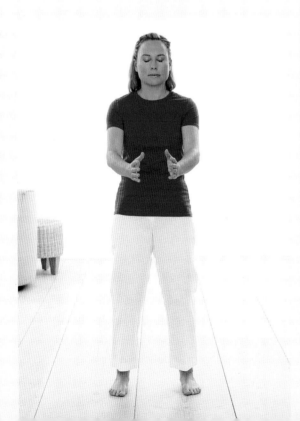

chi face wash

1 Warm up the palms of your hands by rubbing them together and generating chi energy. When you feel significant warmth, use your hands to 'wash' your face with the chi you have generated.

2 Place your palms over your eyes and move them in a circular motion, circling 36 times. Rub your hands together again to regenerate the chi and then rub your hands up and down on the sides of your face 36 times. Let your thumb rub the back of your ears at the same time.

3 Regenerate the chi once more and rub the sides of your nose and the sinus cavities. Rub your hands together again and move down to the throat and pull your throat with alternate hands 36 times.

4 Rub your hands together for the last time, then cover your face and feel the penetrating and relaxing chi.

the qualities of chi

The primary quality of chi is that it is always in motion, in a perpetual state of flux or change. It accumulates, disperses, expands and contracts. Although it surrounds and animates everything, it is not a free-flowing energy separate from reality. Rather, it is subject to the laws of our universe, which the Chinese call li, meaning 'patterns' or 'principles'.

If we have an orange, for example, we can separate it into its pattern or li (its round shape and typical size), and its expression of chi (a combination of its ingredients such as fibre, water and sugar molecules, and vitamin C). This is an example of chi energy manifesting into matter and taking the li or pattern of an orange.

patterns and states

Chi manifests in patterns according to the laws of the universe, like the movement of clouds across the sky.

Another aspect of chi is that it moves in an orderly fashion. It does not move indiscriminately here and there, but travels in waves and patterns, like the wind, the rising and setting of the sun, the seasons, the trees or the clouds. Chi also exists in many different states, in the same way that matter can exist as a solid, a liquid or a vapour. For example, electricity can be a current or a field, and so can chi. Chi can function as an energy field when in the form of 'Wei Chi', the body's defensive energy, or it can function as a current as it flows through the body's meridians, the invisible pathways of chi in the body.

feeling the flow

When you begin to work with chi energy and become more sensitive to its existence, you may begin to feel it moving through your body. You might experience a tingling sensation, a tension along its pathways, or a spreading warmth as it flows from one meridian to the next. You may also feel when it is stagnant or stuck, which can manifest as pain and stiffness. You may begin to discern a tenderness or empty feeling in certain points along your meridians depending on the condition of your chi.

Although chi is an energy, it does not move like lightning or an electrical current through your body, but in a gentler, more flowing fashion, similar to the flow of blood and lymph.

A Taoist priest leads a ceremony at a ritual altar with monks in assistance.

spiritual dimensions

In Asian cultures, chi is also seen as a spiritual force. Mystics throughout time have identified different planes of existence that correlate with higher states of consciousness. The Taoist meditation practices that rely on the breath and the intentional circulation of chi, not only fine-tune the physical body, but also induce higher vibrations of energy. These vibrations of energy can lead to higher states of consciousness and profound spiritual realizations. Taoist meditation practices open you to the presence of the Tao so that you will eventually merge and become one with it (see pages 110–125).

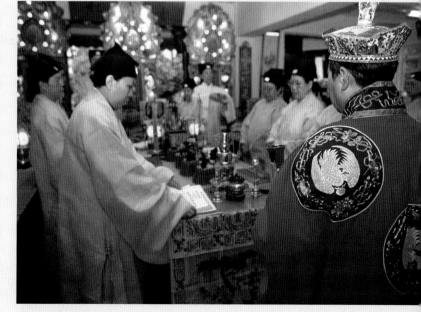

chi and the dance of yin and yang

The Eastern concept of yin and yang is essential to understanding chi. According to the Chinese, chi manifests as yin and yang, that is, through the relationship of opposites. Through exploring yin and yang we can further understand how chi functions and flows in the body and in the universe.

symbolism

Originally, yin and yang were used to describe the ever-changing sunny and shady sides of a mountain.

The meaning of yin and yang is inherent in the famous black and white T'ai Chi symbol, sometimes also depicted in dark blue and red. The circle around the outside represents the Wu Chi mentioned in the Taoist story of the birth of the universe (see page 12). It is the pregnant void from which everything emerges, also known as the Tao, the Single Principle, the Great Void, the Great Ultimate or the One Supreme Unity.

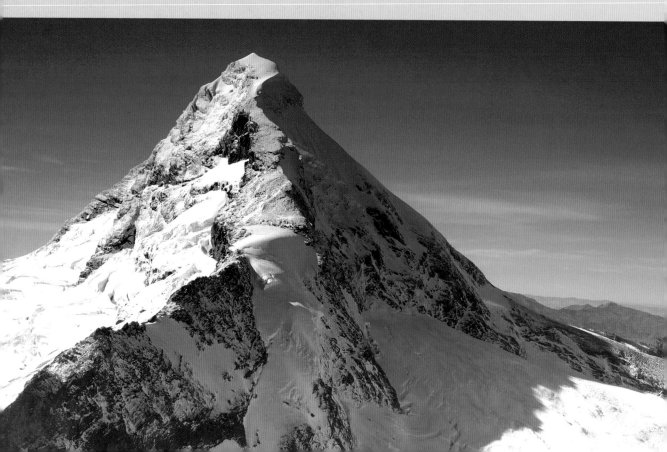

opposite principles

This great void or Tao is then divided into two opposite energy principles that interact with each other: yin (the black half) and yang (the white half). Finally, within each half is a small circle representing its opposite aspect. This is a reminder that nothing is or ever remains absolutely one thing. There is always light within the dark, as in the twinkling stars in the night sky, dark within the light, as in the shadows cast by the sun's rays.

coming to terms with the shadow

On a personal level, we struggle with our dark aspects. Along with our wonderful positive qualities, we carry a shadow made up of those negative aspects of our personality – our jealousy, anger and fear – that make us three-dimensional and fully human. The small circle in each side of the yin/yang symbol reminds us that extreme yang will eventually become yin, and vice versa. Night will turn into day, and even extreme anger can transform into profound love. The curving line represents the continuous interaction and movement between the dark and the light, the negative and positive, and male and female. All is change; nothing is ever static nor remains the same. Through its dance of the opposites of yin and yang, chi manifests as everything.

changing energies

Originally, the terms yin and yang were used to describe the sunny and shady sides of a mountain. Because the sun is rising, moving across the sky and setting, the sunny and shady sides continuously change. The symbol captures this dynamic quality of the movement of light and dark, and the interaction of yin and yang. It also represents the dynamic, changing quality of chi energy. The side of the mountain that is sunnier, hotter, louder, dryer and more active is considered yang, and the side that is cooler, darker, wetter and less active is considered yin. The yang principle is more outwards, male (without regard to gender), more expansive, upward-moving, active and relating to the sun. The yin principle is considered more downwards-moving, lunar, cold, dark, passive, submissive and female, again without regard to gender. Both aspects are necessary for a healthy, balanced life.

yin and yang characteristics

The following list of opposites will help you start to think about how chi manifests as both yin and yang.

Yang	Yin
Active	Passive
Hot	Cold
Dry	Wet
Life	Death
Summer	Winter
Male	Female
Day	Night
Light	Dark
Sun	Moon
Dominant	Submissive
Creative	Receptive
Front	Back
Right	Left
Hard	Soft
Expansive	Contracting
Upwards	Downwards

the qualities of yin and yang

Dark and light, or yin and yang coexist on the planet at the same time.

When thinking about how chi manifests as yin and yang, it is important to remember that yin and yang do not exclude each other. They are not rigid, static categories since nothing is completely yin or yang (see pages 16–17). In fact, yin and yang are interdependent and cannot exist separately. Light cannot exist without darkness. Life cannot exist without death.

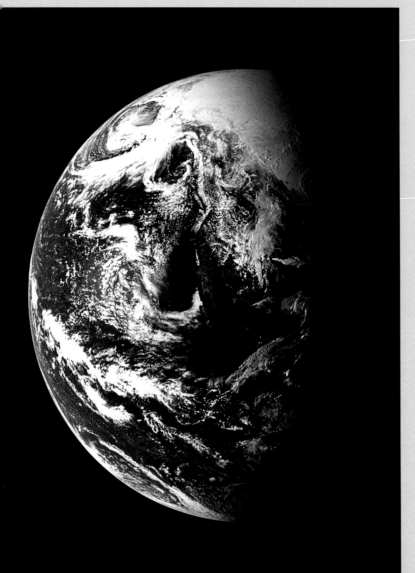

duality and relativity

In addition, yin and yang are always relative. For example, we could say that the air temperature today is either hot or cold. However, hot could mean a scorching desert temperature or simply a warmer temperature in relation to the cooler night air. In other words, within each duality there are always infinite nuances and subdivisions.

Other qualities of yin and yang are that they both consume and support each other. They are often held in balance, so as one increases, the other decreases. When it comes to physical health, mental and emotional states, and the environment around us, imbalances occur. When our bodies are too yin we correct this by bringing it more to yang. If the body is too cold we apply warming remedies like extra layers of clothing. If we find we are too yang and aggressive, we can balance this by trying to express the more yin, passive and nurturing aspects of our character.

transformation

Yin and yang can transform into one another; night changes into day, warmth eventually cools and life changes to death. However, even this transformation is relative. As we know from observing satellite images of the earth, night and day coexist on our planet earth at the same time.

embrace paradox

Through exploring the concept of yin and yang, we can learn to reject rigid states of mind and embrace paradox. The terms 'both/and' rather than 'either/or' are inherent in the yin/yang symbol. For example, a situation can be both good and bad simultaneously, as in a bittersweet meeting with an ex-lover. We may be happy to see our old flame, but we may have a tinge of sadness at the loss. The ability to embrace paradox, to accept the good and the bad, the yin and yang in every situation, is one aspect of emotional and psychological maturity.

balancing yin and yang

One of the biggest misconceptions about yin and yang is that if something is yin it is thought to have less chi energy and if it is yang it has more. But the nature of yin is that it collects chi energy and doesn't expend it whereas yang expends chi energy. Think of a more yin person sitting quietly in the audience while a more yang person performs on stage gesturing energetically and singing in a loud voice. The more yin, receptive person sitting quietly, is gathering chi energy from the singer and conserving his or her own chi, whereas the yang person is expending it. Our fast-paced yang lives need yin down-time to replenish and renew our chi energy. A major aspect of working with chi energy is balancing yin and yang, in our bodies and our lives.

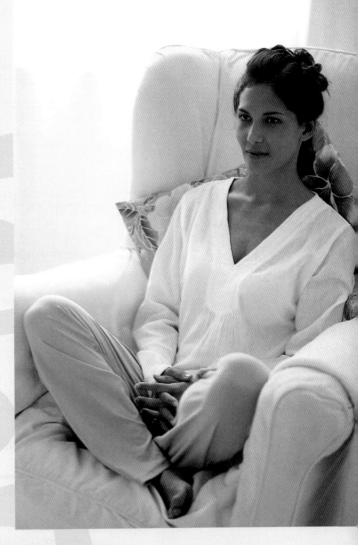

In a fast-paced yang world it is important to embrace quiet yin time to replenish chi energy.

an introduction to Taoism

The concepts of chi, yin and yang, Wu Chi and Tao are all part of Taoism, one of the great religious and philosophical traditions of China. Taoism has had an enormous influence on medicine, the arts and social and intellectual life in China for more than 3,000 years.

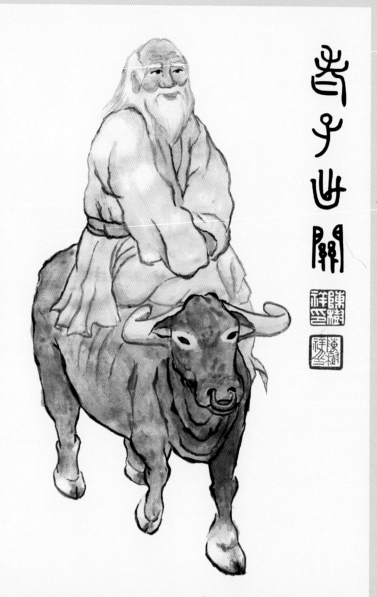

Taoist philosophers

During the classical period of Taoism, between the 8th and 3rd centuries BCE, lived two of the greatest Taoist philosophers — Lao-tzu and Chuang-tzu. Around 600 BCE, Lao-tzu wrote the text *Tao-te ching*, which roughly translated to English is 'The Canon of the Path of Virtue'. Lao-tzu promoted an idea of the universe based on the concept of Tao, the One Supreme Unity. He also introduced the idea of Wu Wei or non-action, and the concept of harmonious, balanced living in tune with nature and the laws of the universe.

Lao-tzu struggled with and eventually rode the bull, representing his victory over negative reactive emotions.

self-transformation

Chuang-tzu wrote the famous text *Chang-tzu* sometime in the 4th or 3rd century BCE. He extended Lao-tzu's thought and introduced the idea of self-transformation, embodied in the practice of T'ai Chi and Chi Kung. He emphasized the dynamic and ever-changing aspect of reality, and felt it was imperative that we transcend the dualities of existence and experience the Tao itself, where all dualities resolve into unity. He revealed that much of the meaning of the universe is bound up in paradox or apparent contradictions — what appears to be yin and yang, for example. He taught that the universe is, in actuality, the Tao, the unity of all things. If we identify with this unity, we no longer fear death or life, and achieve profound tranquillity. Like Buddha before him, he spoke of the possibility of a great awakening — the experience of the Tao as enlightenment.

working with the universe

The goal of Taoists is to be in alignment with the Tao, the Great Void, or the One Supreme Unity, the non-being underlying all being, the unnameable force behind all things, sometimes called the womb from which all things are born and to which all things return. The Tao keeps the universe balanced and ordered. Nature is thought to be a manifestation of the Tao. The flow of chi and the dance of yin and yang are the essential energies of action and existence. For Taoists, the universe works harmoniously. To exert your will against the natural order of things, to try to swim against the current, causes you to disrupt the harmony in yourself and the harmony of the world.

Herbal teas can promote balanced chi and are an important aspect of Taoist healing arts.

Taoism, chi and immortality

Taoists believe that human beings are a microcosm of the universe and by understanding ourselves we can gain knowledge of the universe. The body and the universe are said to be made up of five elements – Water, Fire, Earth, Metal and Wood. The five organ systems correlate with the five elements and the seasons (see *Chi and the five elements*, pages 38–47). The emphasis on nature and the elements, harmony with the seasons and the cyclic flow of chi are examples of Taoist influence on the Chinese view of physical and mental health.

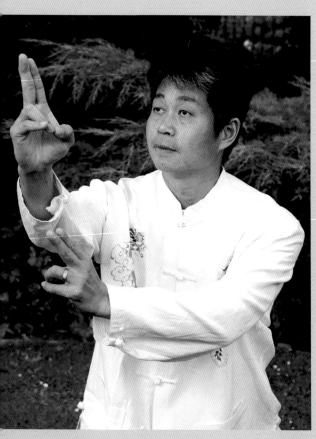

The Taoist ideal was to live an extraordinarily long life, even to strive for immortality. Fantastic tales of Chinese Taoist practitioners said to be hundreds of years old are still told today. The search for elixirs and magical potions to extend their lives led Taoist sages to experiment with a wide variety of plant, animal and mineral elements. Many were discovered to have beneficial and healing properties and are still used widely in China today.

physical practices

Chi-enhancing practices such as Chi Kung, which are used widely in contemporary China and the West to balance and enhance the flow of chi in the body, can also be traced back to the Taoist search for immortality. Chi Kung exercises were based on early Taoist breathing methods and stances designed to purify the body and maintain health.

A person practising Chi Kung to promote the harmonious flow of chi in his body.

Acupressure massage, herbal therapy, acupuncture and the actual transference of chi from healer to patient were part of the healing arts practised in Taoist temples and monasteries in China. Martial arts such as T'ai Chi, Bagua and Xing Yi all have their roots in Taoist practice and rely on the cultivation of internal chi energy rather than outward force.

the three treasures

Taoists believe that humans possess Three Treasures – jing (essence), chi (energy) and shen (spirit).

Jing is stored in the kidneys, but also in the brain, ovaries, semen and bone marrow. It determines your overall vitality, longevity and resistance to illness and disease. There are two kinds of jing – one is the primordial energy that is passed on to you from your parents at conception, it is the energetic counterpart to your DNA and is unique to you. This jing is prenatal energy and governs your growth process. The second type of jing is acquired jing that you obtain through food, which can enhance or magnify your congenital jing. One can never have enough jing.

Chi is the most dynamic and immediate energy of the body, derived from the interaction of yin and yang. Chi has a yang, warming quality that can foster a sense of harmony and wellness. Its counterpart is the blood, which is yin. The blood supports and nurtures chi, while the chi reciprocates by directing blood flow. A healthy person has an abundance of constantly circulating chi, which moves around his or her body. Chi can be strengthened through the intake of food and air, and through exercises like Chi Kung and T'ai Chi.

Shen is one's psyche or spirit. Shen is the energy that rules mental, spiritual and creative activities, and is also said to rule chi. The quality of your spirit will influence the power of your chi flow. If your shen or spirit is weak, it may manifest as anxiety, depression, restlessness or physical illness. Shen can be strengthened through meditation, exercise, good nutrition and herbal remedies.

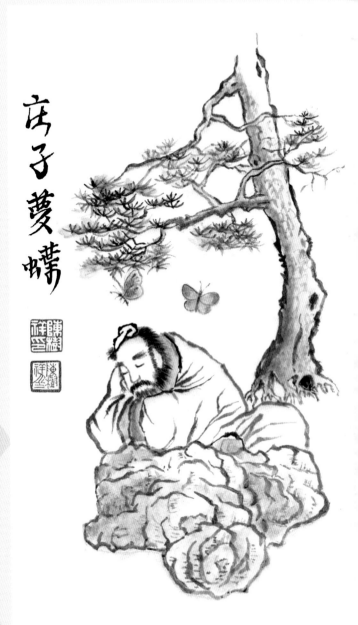

Taoist philosopher Chuang-tzu dreaming his spirit is as free as a butterfly.

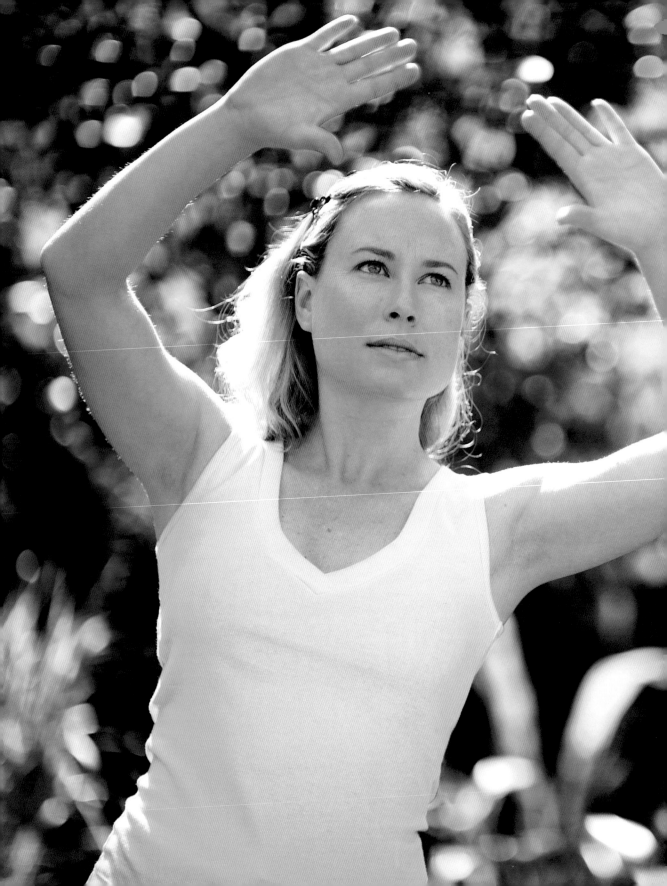

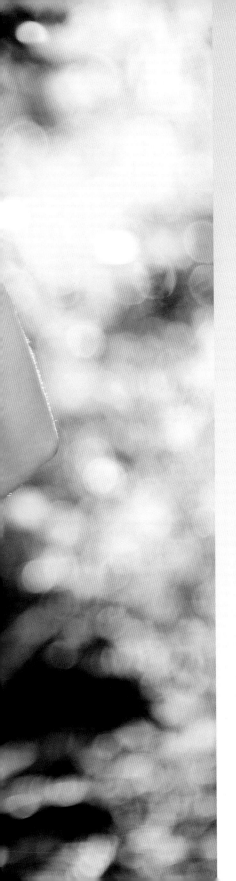

THE HEALING PROMISE OF CHI

The healing promise of chi is that we have the knowledge and ability to work with it – to balance and strengthen it through diet, exercise and meditation – and significantly improve the quality of our lives. The Chinese have created elegant, sophisticated, yet easy-to-learn methods to increase and maintain our energy, health and well-being. We can also work with our chi to support and enhance our spiritual development. Working with chi energy shifts our way of thinking about our bodies away from a physical and mechanical paradigm, towards the holistic and energetic.

mechanical vs energetic views of the body

The modern Western, Newtonian approach to the body emphasizes matter over energy. The body is viewed as a sophisticated collection of systems and parts. Specialists become experts in treating only one aspect – the heart or the lungs or the endocrine system, or the mind and emotions, which are considered separate from the body. The function of a general practitioner is to make an initial diagnosis and then to refer the patient to the correct specialist for further treatment.

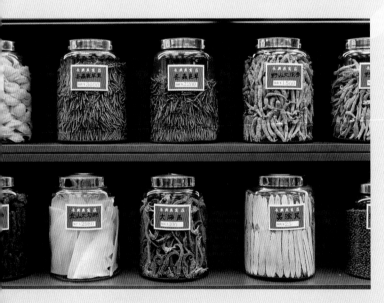

Chinese herbs are powerful remedies for healing illness and balancing chi energy in the body.

treating the once-incurable

Modern medicine is miraculous, life saving and at times positively heroic. Some diseases, such as polio and tuberculosis, and many kinds of infections have been greatly reduced or eradicated through the use of miracle drugs, antibiotics and vaccines. Today, Western scientists are making headway in treating diseases that were previously untreatable, such as Parkinson's disease and diabetes. Clearly, Western medicine, in many ways, has been extraordinarily successful.

But there is much to learn from the Eastern approach to medicine, which considers the body as a whole (including the mind and emotions), and views it as an energetic system rather than a mechanical one. In fact, we need both Eastern and Western approaches for optimal health. If you have a serious illness, applying both Eastern and Western treatments can increase your chance of recovery. Working with your chi through balanced diet, exercise and meditation will help you maintain your health, while Western medicine can provide effective surgical intervention.

integrating east and west

Most Chinese in China do not see traditional Chinese medicine and Western medicine as being in conflict. It is understood that you see a Western doctor if you have an acute illness such appendicitis, but you practise Chi Kung or take Chinese herbs to keep your chi flowing in a healthy way in order to prevent appendicitis, or to recover more quickly from surgery. In China, Western medicine and Chinese medicine are often integrated. For example, at the Shanghai Cancer Hospital, a patient may be seen by a multidisciplinary team and be treated concurrently with surgery, radiation and acupuncture to balance chi flow, modern drugs and a traditional herbal formula. As another example, most Western hospitals now offer T'ai Chi or Chi Kung classes as part of their in-patient and community health programmes.

The Eastern view is not one of heroic intervention but of preventive medicine. When disease does occur, if it is not acute, the goal is to not treat the symptoms but to bring the body back into balance, allowing chi to flow freely throughout the meridian system. A key principle of traditional Chinese medicine is that when chi flows smoothly your internal systems function optimally. Your blood circulation improves, allowing more oxygen and nutrients to be delivered to all areas of the body so it can heal itself more efficiently. Maintaining good chi flow keeps the body, mind and emotions in balance, leading to optimal health.

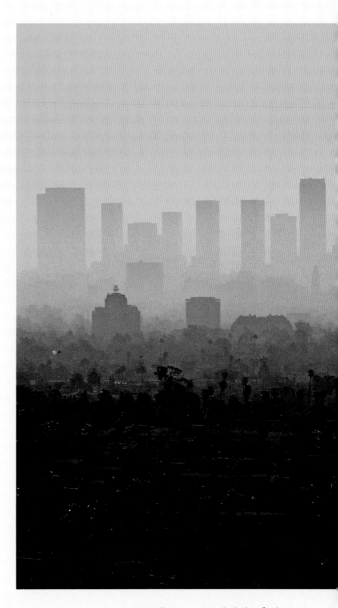

Air pollution, pesticide-laden foods and the pervasive use of toxic chemicals in everyday life stress the body and weaken chi.

resisting negative energies

In today's busy, fast-paced world, we are continually exposed to the everyday stresses of making a living and negotiating our many relationships. We are bombarded by toxins that pollute our food and environment.

When negative energies invade our bodies, through pesticide-laden or unhealthy food, polluted air, external pathogens or stressful situations, blockages are created that impede the flow of chi or chi is weakened, causing a deficiency. If balance is not restored, the normal physiological functioning of the body becomes impaired. When chi is not flowing smoothly, it can result in a lack of vitality, physical pain, reduced mobility, injury, emotional imbalance, rapid ageing or illness.

restoring balance

Acupuncture is the practice of inserting very fine needles in points along the meridians to restore balance and harmony to the body.

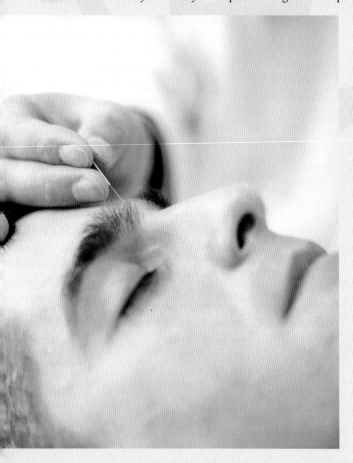

Chinese health practitioners use a variety of techniques to restore a balanced flow of chi through the body. Acupuncture is used to manipulate points or 'gates' to open blocked meridians or to strengthen deficient chi thus restoring balance and harmony. In addition, Chinese doctors use a wide variety of herbs, minerals and animal products made into teas to help open blockages and maintain a smooth flow of chi in the body, so the body, mind and emotions can heal. Breathing exercises, Chi Kung, T'ai Chi and meditation are sometimes recommended to enhance the flow of chi through the body and to help the patient manage his or her own chi. These are the same techniques that Taoist masters have used for thousands of years to achieve spiritual realizations, longevity and a higher quality of life.

treating a headache

A Chinese doctor will not offer you a painkiller, but will conduct an examination to determine the chi imbalance causing your distress. He or she will determine which meridian/organ systems are the source of the headache and bring them back into balance with acupuncture or a herbal remedy. In order to diagnose your imbalance, the doctor will take your pulses (three on each wrist), examine your tongue, the

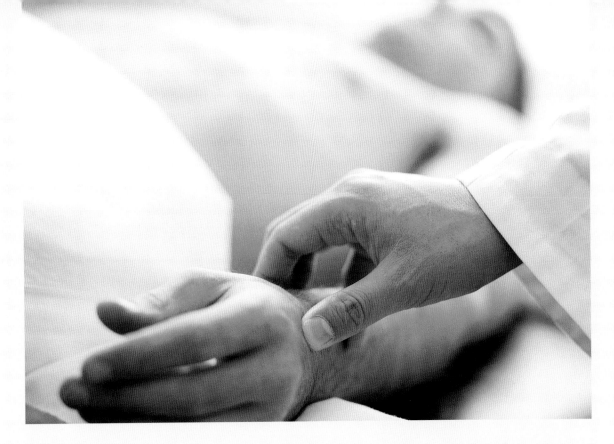

colour of your skin, the condition of your eyes and nails, and take note of your demeanour, mood and body language. The doctor will listen to the quality of your voice.

Chinese doctors assess health by taking multiple pulses on each wrist that correspond to various meridian and organ systems.

Then the doctor will ask him- or herself a series of questions to determine the nature, location and origin of your symptoms. He or she may perform acupuncture using needles inserted in various points along the meridians appropriate for your condition. The practitioner may prescribe dietary changes or Chi Kung exercises for stress relief.

Unlike Western medicine, Chinese medicine is completely holistic and has no 'one size fits all' treatment. If three different patients complain of headaches, the doctor may prescribe entirely different acupuncture points and/or herbs based on the unique physical and emotional imbalance each patient presents. When patients have many different complaints – perhaps a migraine headache, insomnia, pain in the upper right side under the ribs and difficulty with anger – Chinese doctors will treat all symptoms, physical and emotional, as interconnected. The cure for any complaint or set of complaints is to rebalance the flow of chi in the body so that organs, bones or tissues will function properly, and the emotional and spiritual life can be enhanced.

eight principles of Chinese medicine

A Chinese doctor will use the four basic polarities or eight principles to assess a patient. They are basically a series of questions that help to determine the state of the patient's chi energy, and help the practitioner decide how best to rebalance it and restore health to the body.

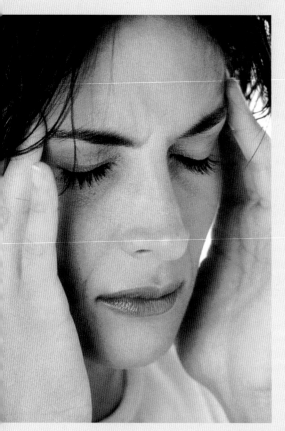

If you have a headache, a Chinese doctor will conduct an examination to determine the chi imbalance.

The doctor will ask if the symptoms are: excess or deficient; hot or cold; yin or yang; and internal or external.

- If you have excess chi or your chi is stagnant or congested, you may experience swelling, pain or throbbing. If your chi is deficient, you may have weakness, fatigue, a pale complexion or wounds that won't heal.
- Your symptoms may be identified as hot if you have a fever, a flushed complexion and dehydration; or they may be identified as cold if you have a runny nose, diarrhoea and a slow pulse.
- If the location of your symptoms is deep in your body, relating to your internal organs or blood, or if you have swelling, 'dampness' or excess fluids, then your symptoms are considered yin. If your complaint has to do with your muscles or skin, or 'dryness' and a scarcity of fluids, then your symptoms are yang in nature.
- If the origin of your symptoms is the weather or exposure to germs, it is external. External symptoms are also at the surface of the body: the skin, muscles and mucous membranes. Most common illnesses, such as colds or flu, allergies, muscle and joint aches, headaches and skin rashes, are considered external symptoms. If your symptoms are from an imbalance in your organs, hormones, stress or your emotions, the origin is considered internal.

To make things a little more complicated, your symptoms can manifest in combinations. But try not to feel overwhelmed. Assessing your body in this way is more an art than a science. If you work with the principles, over time they will teach you to pay closer attention to your physical body, the state of your chi energy and the nuances of how you feel. Working with the principles will help you practise better self-care.

assessing your cold or flu using the eight principles

As we all know, the common cold or flu can manifest in many different ways and move through different phases. The Chinese approach is to apply the appropriate remedy for whatever phase the virus is in using the eight principles.

1 Excess or deficient: Ask yourself these questions. Is your cold or flu manifesting excess – red face, red eyes, fever, sore throat, muscles aches or coarse breathing? Or is it manifesting a deficiency – loss of energy, pale complexion, slow weak pulse or loose stools.

2 Hot or cold: Ask yourself if your symptoms are hot – fever, swollen glands, dry mouth and increased thirst, no sweating, coloured phlegm? Or cold – chills, cold extremities, runny nose, slow pulse, pallor, spontaneous sweating?

3 Yin or yang: Ask yourself if your cold started with a feeling of losing energy, a slow or weak pulse and a pale complexion – in which case you probably have a yin constitution. If it started with an aggressive response, such as a scratchy or sore throat, muscles aches and swollen glands, you probably have a more yang constitution.

4 External or internal: Cold and flu are considered external in nature.

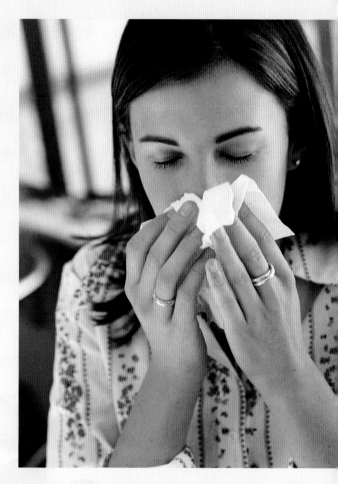

In the Chinese system, a cold or flu may manifest yin or yang symptoms and will be treated accordingly.

the benefits of working with chi

Chi is free and it is everywhere. The whole universe, ourselves and all animate and inanimate things are bathed in it, and are actually made of chi. Your body is kept alive by the flow of chi. The good news is that you can do a lot to enhance your health and well-being by becoming conscious of the existence of chi and learning how it functions.

Finding a good Chinese medical practitioner and having a professional assessment and treatment is one of the best things you can do for your health. But there are simple methods you can use on your own to manage your chi energy and enhance your health and vitality.

working with chi

You can learn how chi flows through your body, and how yin and yang manifest in the meridians and organ systems and in the food you ingest. By adjusting what you eat you can enhance chi flow and balance the yin and yang energies on your bodies. You can learn how the state of your chi influences your health and emotions. By learning simple massage techniques, Chi Kung and T'ai Chi exercises, meditation and dietary practices, you can begin to experience a profound improvement in your daily life, and gain access to greater energy and vitality. Working with chi and meditation will help bring you to a higher state of consciousness.

Working with your chi makes you more conscious of the fact that you are a being made of light and energy. You can become more responsible for your own health and well-being. Rather than giving up your power to medical professionals, you can begin to take your health into your own hands. In the following chapters we will learn ways to manage chi. But first, there is more to learn about chi, including how we gather it, the four kinds of chi and how chi behaves in disharmony.

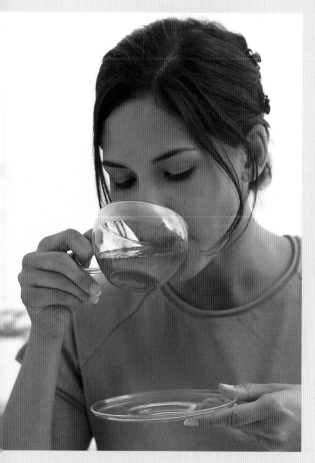

Drinking herbal teas appropriate for your constitution is an effective way to balance your chi energy.

your body's three sources of chi

According to Chinese medicine, there are three sources of chi energy in your body. You gather chi from:

- your parents at conception
- food you eat and liquids you drink
- air you breathe.

The chi from your parents is stored in your kidneys. Chi that you take in from your environment through nutrition and respiration is processed by your organs, and stored and circulated throughout your body through your meridians, the pathways of chi. When the flow of chi is impeded or depleted in some way, you will experience emotional and physical imbalance that manifests in a variety of symptoms. Some will be minor and others may eventually lead to serious illness. On the other hand, when your chi is flowing freely and nourishing your body and mind, you can experience extraordinary health and vitality.

One of the three sources of chi energy comes from the air we breathe.

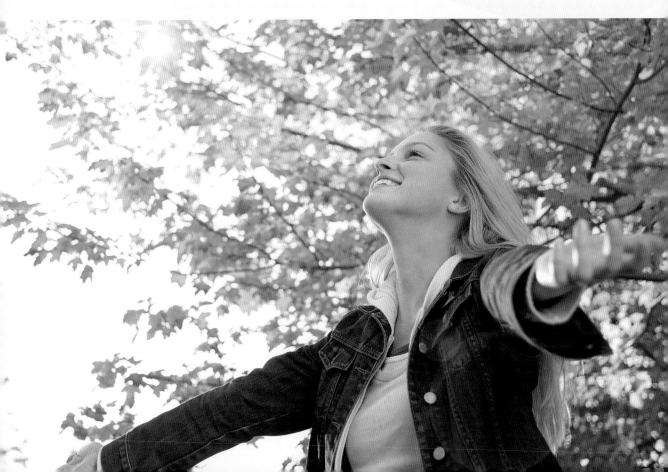

the four kinds of chi

There are many kinds of chi, but the main four found in the body are original chi, pectoral chi, nourishing chi and defensive chi.

original chi

Also called kidney chi, this most important chi is the one you were born with and that you receive from your parents. The growth and development of your body, and the function of your organs depend on your original chi. When your original chi is sufficient, your organs will function well and your constitution will be good. However, if your original chi is deficient due to a congenital defect or improper nutrition as a baby, your whole body will become weakened. This can lead to slow growth and development, a compromised immune system and a fearful nature. Chronic diseases can also deplete original chi. This chi cannot be created but is enhanced and supported by the other three forms of chi.

Original chi, or pre-birth chi, is inherited from your parents and enhanced by the other forms of chi.

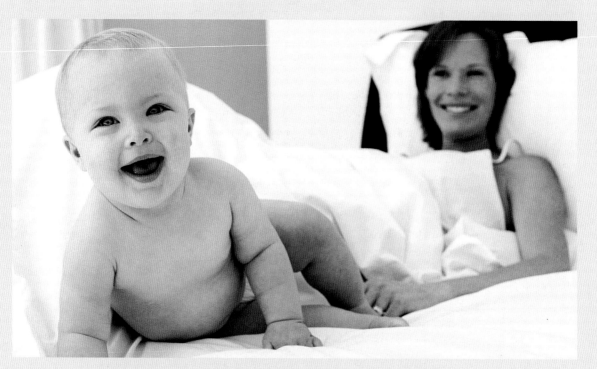

pectoral chi

Also called great chi, pectoral chi accumulates in your chest area. Pectoral chi is generated by the food you eat, which is transformed by your spleen and the fresh air you inhale. Pectoral chi assists your lungs in breathing. If you speak clearly, have a strong voice and good respiration, you have strong pectoral chi. If you have slurred speech, a feeble voice, shallow breathing or shortness of breath, you have deficient pectoral chi. Pectoral chi assists your heart in pumping and regulating the flow of blood. When it is sufficient, you will feel emotionally balanced, your pulse will be strong and your heart will beat with a steady rhythm. If your pectoral chi is deficient, your pulse will be fast, irregular or weak. With deficient pectoral chi you may have cold hands and feet, low energy and move with difficulty.

nourishing chi

Also known as acquired chi, this is the chi that flows in your blood vessels and, as you can tell from its name, is rich in nutrients. Like pectoral chi, it is formed by the intake of food and fresh air, and supports your original chi. The main functions of nourishing chi are to create blood and to nourish the whole body. Nourishing chi absorbs nutrition and body fluids from digested food and carries it to the vessels to form blood. All of your organs, meridians and tissues depend on nourishing chi in order to function. If your nourishing chi is sufficient you will be in good physical and emotional health. Digestive problems, bowel problems and diseases of the blood are related to deficient nourishing chi.

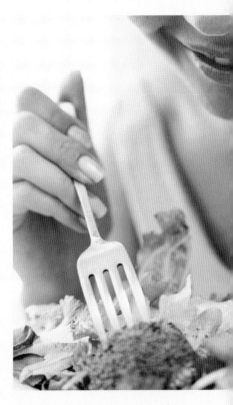

The water we drink, the food we eat and the air we breathe generate pectoral and nourishing chi.

defensive chi

This chi defends your body and supports your immune system. Like pectoral and nourishing chi, defensive chi is created from nutritious food and fresh air. There are three main functions of defensive chi: guarding the surface of the body against invasion by pathogens; keeping a relatively constant body temperature by controlling the opening and closing of the pores; and adjusting the excretion of sweat and nourishing the organs, bowels, muscles, skin and hair. If you catch colds easily, suffer from fever or chills or take a long time to recover from illness, you may have deficient defensive chi.

the three states of chi

According to traditional Chinese medicine, chi circulates in the body along its own energetic pathways called channels or meridians, in the same way that blood circulates in the arteries and veins. The one exception is defensive chi that functions as a 'field' and circulates between the skin and the flesh to protect the body, and as a current as it moves along the meridians. Chi is also present in the blood and is said to be the energy that animates it and moves it along. Whatever kind of chi it is, it will be in one of three states – harmony, deficiency or stagnation.

When your chi is sufficient, balanced and functioning in a harmonious way, you will be in relatively good health, and have the energy and vitality to work and enjoy life. Your mental state will be balanced and you will be able to negotiate the inevitable stresses of life. If your chi is deficient or stagnant, you may not feel very well and possibly have a variety of symptoms or complaints.

signs of harmonious chi

Absence of pain
Happiness
Contentment
Good stamina
Restful sleep
Vibrant energy
Creativity
Productivity
Normal body temperature

signs of deficient and stagnant chi

Feeling cold
Feeling weak
Persistent fatigue
Sexual or menstrual problems
Frequent colds or flu
Allergies
Anger, fear, worry, mania
Depression or anxiety
Insomnia
Illness or disease
Lethargy
Digestive/bowel problems
Procrastination
Low or high body temperature

assessing your chi

Now that you have read about the four kinds of chi, it is time to determine which ones you feel are strong in you and which, if any, are compromised.

1 Set aside some time when you won't be disturbed to think about your chi. For example, were you born with congenital heart disease or any other genetically inherited condition? Do you have digestive problems, a poor diet, insomnia, or do you get colds often? There are no right or wrong answers and a condition may be influenced by more than one kind of chi. Simply thinking of your own body in terms of the four kinds of chi will help you make the shift from a mechanical Western view of the body to an energetic Eastern one.

2 Write down how you feel right now, physically, mentally and emotionally. Try to be as thorough and honest as you can be. Note in what ways you feel in good health, physically, mentally and spiritually. If you come up with some negative symptoms or feelings, instead of thinking of them in traditional Western terms, i.e. I have an infection, or I need an anti-depressant, begin to think of those symptoms as having to do with the state of your chi.

3 Review material in this chapter – the origin of chi, the eight principles of chi, the four kinds of chi and the states of chi – to help you in this mental shift from a mechanical view of the body to an energetic one. Create a journal for assessing your chi.

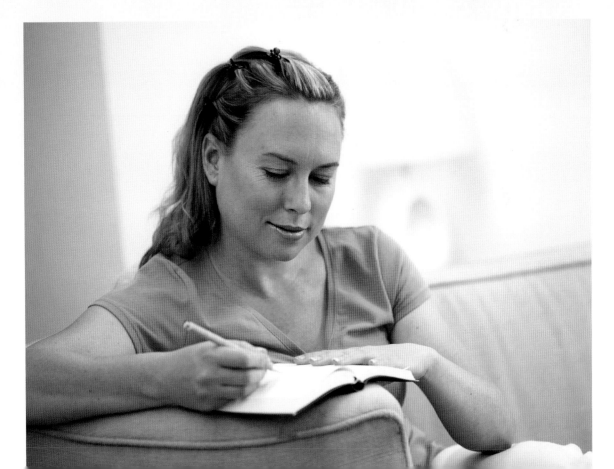

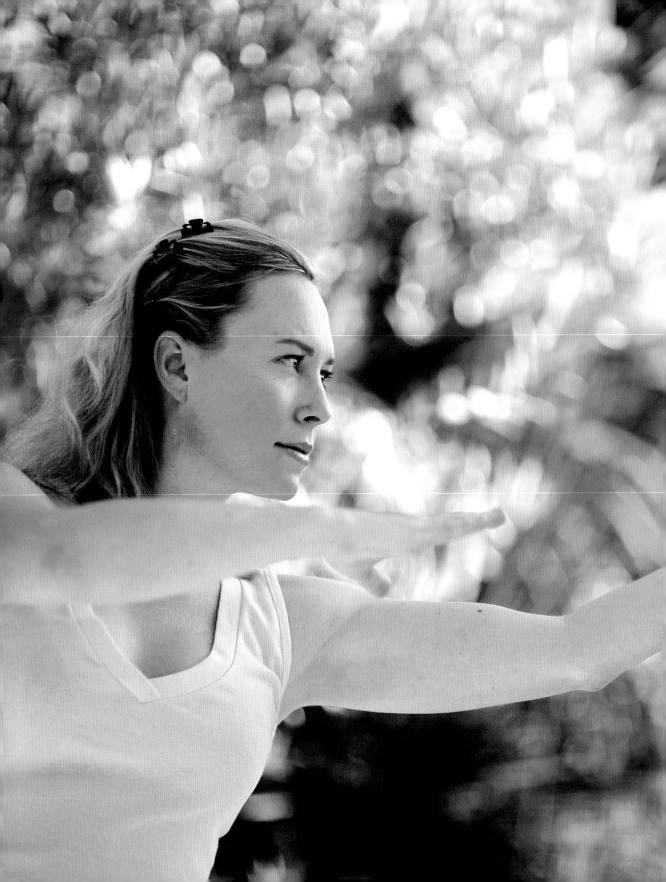

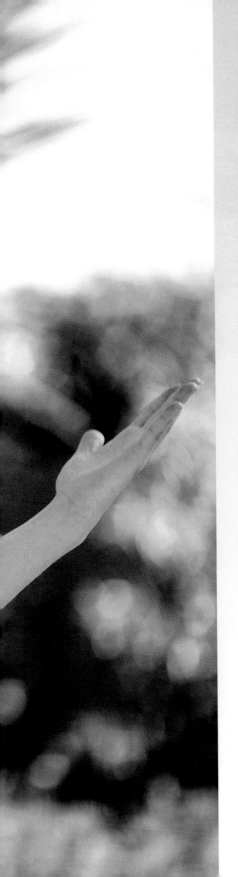

CHI AND THE FIVE ELEMENTS

Taoists believe that the universe and by extension, the body, are made up of five elements: Water, Fire, Earth, Metal and Wood. The five elements provide another way to understand the behaviour of chi and how it affects your health and your life. In this chapter we will begin to see how understanding the five elements or five phases will expand your understanding of how chi moves and manifests in the body. It will also give you more tools for managing your chi, keeping your body balanced and in good health.

the five element system

Five thousand years ago Chinese physicians developed a poetic yet practical approach to understanding the universe and the process of healing, and called it the Five Element System. This system helps you understand how chi moves through the body, who you are, and why you feel and behave the way you do.

The Chinese believe that the five elements – Wood, Fire, Earth, Metal and Water – govern the physical, emotional and spiritual reality of human beings in the same way that they regulate growth and change in the natural world. Each of the elements has a unique quality and everyone favours one or two in their physical, mental and emotional make-up.

This chart shows the creation and destruction cycles of the five elements, and how each element relates to the other in the body and the external world.

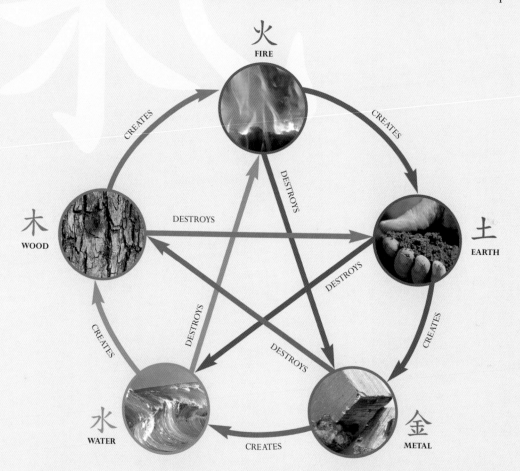

火 FIRE

木 WOOD

土 EARTH

水 WATER

金 METAL

CREATES
CREATES
CREATES
CREATES
CREATES

DESTROYS
DESTROYS
DESTROYS
DESTROYS
DESTROYS

dynamic powers

In the Taoist and Chinese view, the elements are not material substances but dynamic powers or qualities of the universe. In traditional Chinese medicine, each organ system and meridian is governed by one of the five elements. The interdependence of the elements is defined by the generation cycle: Wood feeds Fire, Fire creates Earth, Earth bears Metal, Metal collects Water and Water nourishes Wood; and the destruction cycle: Wood parts Earth, Earth absorbs Water, Water quenches Fire, Fire melts Metal and Metal chops Wood. When one element and its organ/meridian system is weak, the rest will suffer; when one element and its organs are strengthened, others benefit.

the five elements and their associations

	WOOD	FIRE	EARTH	METAL	WATER
Season	Spring	Summer	Late Summer	Autumn	Winter
Weather	Windy	Hot	Humid	Dry	Cold
Time of day	Morning	Midday	Afternoon	Evening	Night
Yin organs	Liver	Heart	Spleen	Lungs	Kidney
Yang organs	Gall bladder	Small intestine	Stomach	Large intestine	Bladder
Tissue	Muscles, tendons	Blood vessels	Flesh	Skin	Bones
Sensory organs	Eyes	Tongue	Mouth	Nose	Ears
Senses	Sight	Speech	Touch	Taste, smell	Hearing
Bodily fluid	Tears	Perspiration	Saliva, lymph	Mucus	Urine
Expression	Nails	Complexion	Lips	Body hair	Head hair
Colour	Green	Red	Yellow	White	Blue, black
Behaviour	Controlling	Crying	Worrying	Coughing	Shaking
Emotion	Anger	Joy	Compassion	Grief	Fear
Tone of voice	Loud, shouting	Laughing	Singing	Whining	Groaning
Spirit	Soul, vision	Consciousness	Intelligence	Instinct	Will to live
Mental activity	Planning	Integration	Reflection	Concentration	Meditation
Energy	Spiritual	Psychological	Physical	Vital	Ancestral
Dream	Forest, trees	Fire, laughter	Music, singing	Flying	Drowning

Wood

The Wood element controls the liver and gall bladder. It nourishes Fire and is overcome by excess Metal.

If you are a Wood person, you may have a bold, commanding personality. You are tenacious like a tree sinking its roots deep into the ground. You have vision and insight and enjoy planning ahead. You make decisions easily. You have an evenly proportioned hand, with many lines on the palms and fingers. When in good health, your body is muscular, athletic and well proportioned.

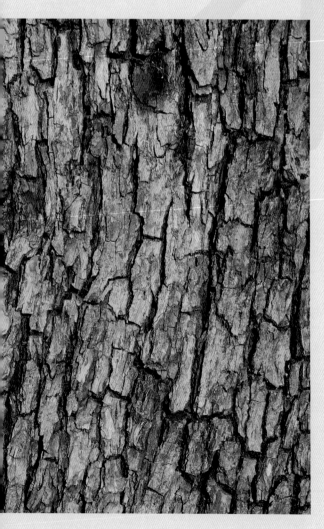

excess Wood chi

Wood controls the liver and gall bladder organ and meridian systems. When you have an excess of liver or gall bladder chi, you may have rigid or cracked fingernails, and muscular tension and spasms, usually in the head, neck and shoulders. You may have frequent headaches, visual problems, dizziness, ringing in the ears, menstrual irregularities, high blood pressure, muscle or eye twitches, and tingling and numbness in your extremities. Easily agitated, you are inflexible and prone to shouting and violent outbursts. Others see you as a workaholic, insensitive and self-destructive.

deficient Wood chi

If your liver or gall bladder chi is deficient you may experience insomnia, lethargy and lack of energy. You may have digestive problems, food sensitivities and allergies of all kinds. Anxiety unrelated to any situation and restless nervous energy are a sign of deficient Wood chi. You may be indecisive and suffer from feelings of shame. Your creative energy may feel blocked, and you may feel stuck and unable to move. Problems with addictions to alcohol, tobacco, sugar, coffee or recreational drugs are often a sign of deficient Wood chi, as are depression and frustration.

Fire

If you are a Fire person, you love to be with people and you cherish your relationships. You are energetic, warm-hearted and emotional. You are passionate, enthusiastic, optimistic and love sensual pleasures. Laughter comes easily to you. You are intuitive and empathetic. Your hands have long, flexible fingers with the small finger bent inward. You have a graceful, willowy body, with a long neck and delicate features.

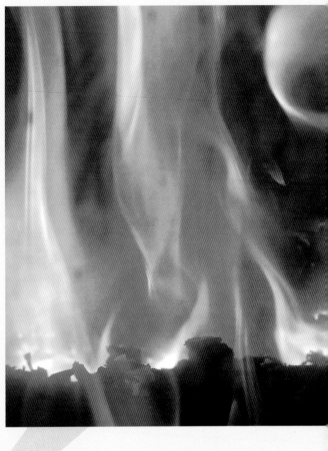

excess Fire chi

Fire controls the heart and small intestine organ and meridian system. When your heart or small intestine chi is in excess, you may have excess perspiration, a tendency to overheat or have hot flashes. A flushed complexion or skin eruptions may occur. You may have heart palpitations, angina, an erratic pulse or irregular heart beat. You may have sleep disturbances or disturbing dreams. Other symptoms are stuttering, strained or rapid speech or hoarseness. You may be restless, agitated or manic. Mood swings, inappropriate, loud and annoying laughter, and irrational thought patterns are also signs.

The Fire element controls the heart and small intestine. It nourishes the Earth and can be overcome by excess Water.

deficient Fire chi

Deficient heart, small intestine chi may manifest as shallow breathing or a tendency to hold your breath. You may have an ashen complexion, rashes or eczema and periods of light-headedness if you get nervous or excited. You may have depressed sexual energy and low blood pressure and perhaps congestive heart failure. You have an intense need to be accepted by others. When it comes to love, you have poor judgement and others find you emotionally unstable. You are forgetful and have difficulty concentrating or thinking logically.

Earth

If you are an Earth person, you are naturally nurturing and caring. You are tolerant, patient and forgiving. You create home, relationship and work situations that are comfortable and stable. Your hand is short with thick fingers, a square palm and flat nails. You have broad, rounded hips and shoulders, smooth skin and dominant mouth and lips.

excess Earth chi

Earth controls the spleen and stomach organ and meridian systems. When your spleen or stomach chi is in excess, your arms and legs feel heavy. If female, you may have PMS, a heavy menstrual flow or fibroid tumours. Your metabolism is sluggish and you gain weight easily. Other symptoms are ulcers and hypothyroidism. You have difficulty with boundaries and others may experience you as meddling. You worry obsessively and your positive nurturing aspect turns into smothering over-protectiveness.

The Earth element controls the spleen and stomach. It nourishes Metal and can be overcome by excess Wood.

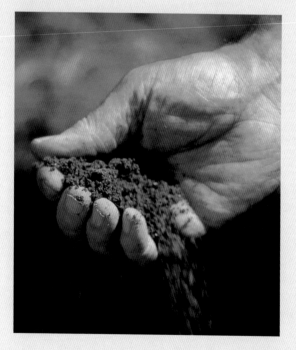

deficient Earth chi

When your spleen and stomach chi is deficient, it may have started in your childhood. If your emotional attachments were ruptured or lacking, you may have deep feelings of inadequacy and have problems taking care of yourself. Deficiency leads to obesity, bloating, loose stools and poor muscle tone. Your limbs, joints and muscles may ache. You may have arthritis, varicose veins, haemorrhoids and a tendency to bruise easily. You crave sugar, carbohydrates and sweetened caffeinated beverages. Blood sugar disturbances such as diabetes or hypoglycaemia may be in your future. You worry obsessively and want to rescue others from their problems while at the same time not being able to solve your own. You feel inadequate and lonely and are needy in relationships. You have difficulty starting projects.

Metal

If you are a Metal person, you are attracted to beauty, symmetry, art, philosophy and the higher truths. You have high moral standards, a keen aesthetic sense and a love of learning. Your hands are long with long palms and square-shaped nails, and you may be double-jointed. You have long arms and legs and your shoulders are narrow. You have small bones and chiselled features. Your nose is most prominent.

excess Metal chi

Metal governs the lung and large intestine. When lung and large intestine chi is in excess, you will have stiff, tight muscles and an awkward posture and movement. Sinus infections are common. Your skin may be very dry, along with your hair, nails and lips. You may have eczema, psoriasis and acne, along with intestinal problems such as colitis, constipation and irritable bowel syndrome. You are formal, emotionally distant, critical and judgemental. You have rituals and an obsession with order and cleanliness. You may collect stamps, coins or other objects.

deficient Metal chi

Metal is about rhythm and order. When your Metal chi is deficient, you become confused and disorganized. You may have congestion, difficulty breathing and a tight chest, along with bronchial spasms or asthma caused by allergies. Moles, warts and cracked, dry nails are common. Because your immune function is compromised, you may have frequent colds and flu or chronic fatigue syndrome. Emotionally, you are numb. You have low self-esteem and you hold on to grief. You have an acute fear of failure and phobias, possibly agoraphobia. Your house is filled with clutter and junk.

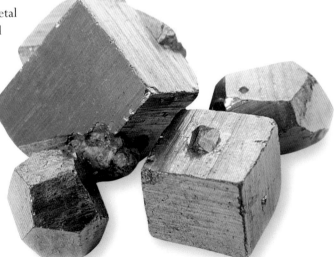

The Metal element controls the lungs and large intestine, nourishes Water and is overcome by excess Fire.

Water

If your element is Water, like Metal, you are interested in the arts, religion and philosophy, but you are more introspective. You love to contemplate the mysteries and meaning of life. Intellectual and visionary, you like to know how things work, from politics to quantum physics. Your hand is short and fleshy, your nails are thin and your cuticles dark. You have a lean body with wider hips and narrow shoulders. Your ears dominate your face.

excess Water chi

Water governs the bladder and kidney. Excess water chi manifests as bad teeth and gums, sleep problems, bladder and prostate problems and kidney stones. Lumps, tumours and hardening of the arteries are common. Vertigo or dizziness can occur, along with high blood pressure, heart attacks and stroke. You may become antisocial, irritable, cynical and depressed. You may be fanatical and inflexible and suspicious of others' motives. You may also obsess about sex. You demand loyalty and are unforgiving of others. You are opinionated and intolerant of other viewpoints.

deficient Water chi

In deficiency, Water chi can cause a lack of energy, dry, split, thinning or balding hair or prematurely grey hair. Dark circles under the eyes signal a weakness in kidney or adrenal function. You may have lower back pain, cold hands and feet, frequent urination and diminished sex drive. Brittle bones and osteoporosis may be present. Absentmindedness, procrastination and lack of motivation are common, along with paranoia, depression and hopelessness. Everything you do is a chore and nothing seems to matter.

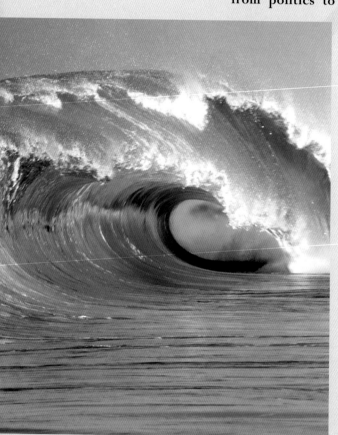

The Water element controls the bladder and kidney. It nourishes Wood and can be overcome by excess Earth.

what element am I?

As you may have noticed, working with chi is much more of an art than a science because chi is always changing, always in motion. Yet, being able to think of your body in an energetic and holistic way can be a relief. Finally, you can make sense of all your physical and emotional symptoms, even your behaviour, because they are all interrelated. In the Chinese system, how you think, feel, look and act can give you clues about your basic nature, as well as the state of your chi and health. Working with chi and the five elements is a wonderful way to begin to understand deeply yourself and others. You may have aspects of each element, but one or two will dominate. The related organ systems are ones for you to monitor and strive to keep healthy.

1 Go over the chart at the beginning of this chapter. You will notice additional ways the elements manifest – through colour preference, tone of voice or the content of dreams. For example, if you are attracted to (or repelled by) dark blue, you may be a Water person or have a water imbalance.

2 Then review the information for each element. Gather five blank sheets of paper, one for each element. Write down characteristics, behaviours and symptoms that seem to describe you under the appropriate element.

3 When you finish your review, notice which elements you favour. This tells you which elements predominate in your body, and the organ and meridian systems to which you need to pay close attention. It will give you a deeper understanding of who you are and how to be true to your own nature. It will also give you a better understanding of the energy patterns that influence the people in your life you know and love.

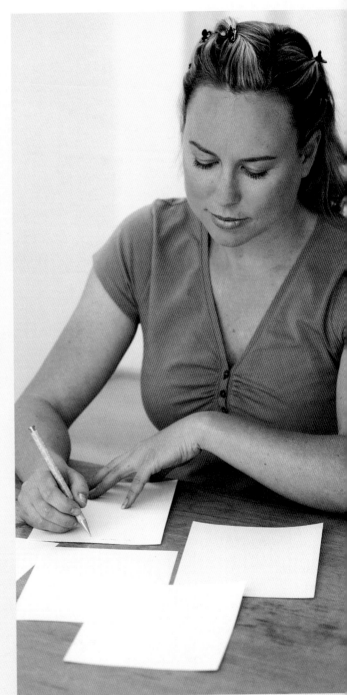

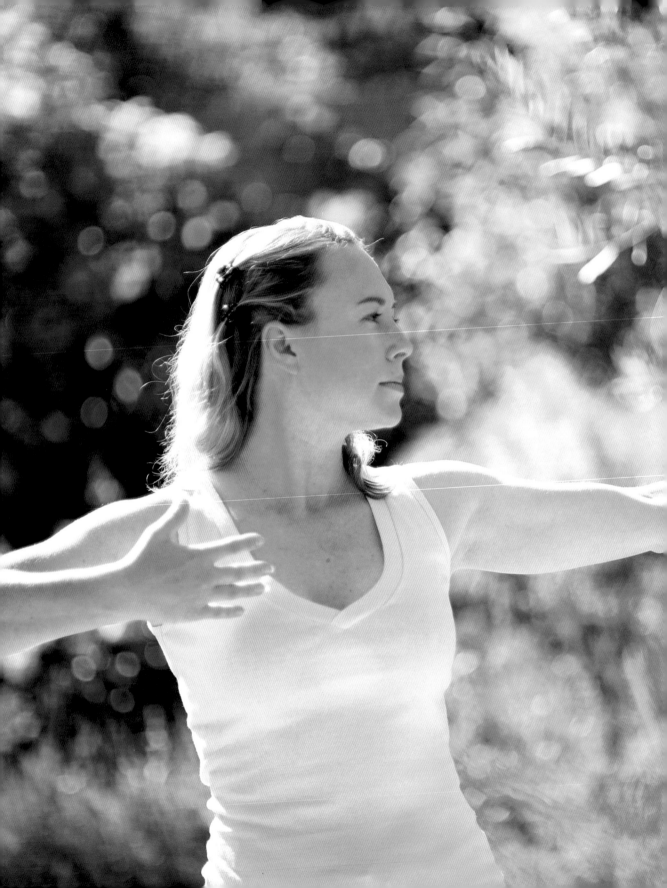

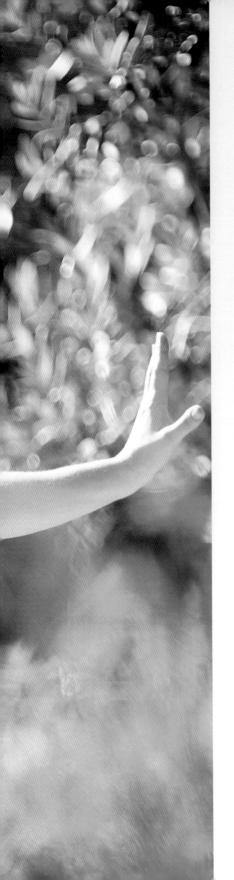

CHI AND YOUR MERIDIANS

Chi travels through your body along a series of interconnected pathways or channels called meridians. Your chi moves in a set order, from one meridian to the next. When blockages or disruptions in the flow of chi energy occur, one or more of your organ systems can become imbalanced, which can result in emotional and/or physical illness.

Along the 12 major meridians are approximately 365 specific points, about the size of a fingertip. These points are the gateways to your chi, and are used both for diagnosing and treating the disruptions in chi flow. Through acupuncture (using very thin small needles) or through acupressure (massaging the appropriate points), chi energy can be stimulated if deficient, or sedated if in excess and brought into balance. Because chi travels in a set order through the meridians, when you target one meridian, the next will also be helped. The Chinese call this the 'mother-child effect'.

the 12 major meridians

The 12 major meridians or channels of chi energy that run through the body are named after the organ or function connected to its energy flow. The same meridians are mirrored or duplicated on the left and right sides of the body. For example, your heart meridian can be found in the same place on your left and right arm. The 12 meridians have an internal and an external pathway. The external pathway of a meridian and its points are what you see on acupuncture charts. The internal pathway constitutes the deeper parts of the meridian where it changes direction and flows 'underground' through the body's cavities and organs, bathing them in life-giving chi.

yin/yang meridians

The six yang meridians are large intestine, stomach, small intestine, bladder, triple warmer and gall bladder. The six yin meridians are lung, spleen, kidney, heart, heart constrictor and liver. There is, of course, no organ named 'heart constrictor' or 'triple warmer' (see page 56). In the Chinese system, heart constrictor describes the function of circulation and triple warmer functions as an energetic thermostat for the upper, middle and lower areas of the torso.

mapping the meridians

When you see an illustration of the human body with all of the meridians and points, it may remind you of an impossibly complicated roadmap. But if you study each meridian separately and begin to trace it on your own or a friend's body, learning the meridian system will become much easier. As you trace a meridian on your own body, you may be able to feel the points as they are often more sensitive to touch than surrounding areas. Where there is excess chi you may feel pain or soreness, where there is deficient chi, the point may feel empty or lacking in energy.

On the following pages, you will be introduced to each meridian in its yin and yang pairs in the order in which the chi flows through your body.

You will learn the element that governs it, its location on the body and the points or gateways to the chi. You will discover each meridian's function and how you might feel if that meridian is in a state of imbalance.

The points on meridians can be stimulated or sedated with massage as well as needles.

meridian massage

Massaging the meridians is an effective alternative to acupuncture with needles. It is possible to massage most of your meridians yourself with the exception of the bladder meridian, which runs the length of your back. (Special massage tools are available online for reaching the bladder points). It is not important to know the points to massage on the meridians. Simply refer to the chart and apply gentle pressure along the meridian, always starting from point number 1, moving in one direction to the ending point. Use your fingers, thumb or palm, and apply gentle pressure along the entire meridian. Remember to massage the meridian on both sides of the body.

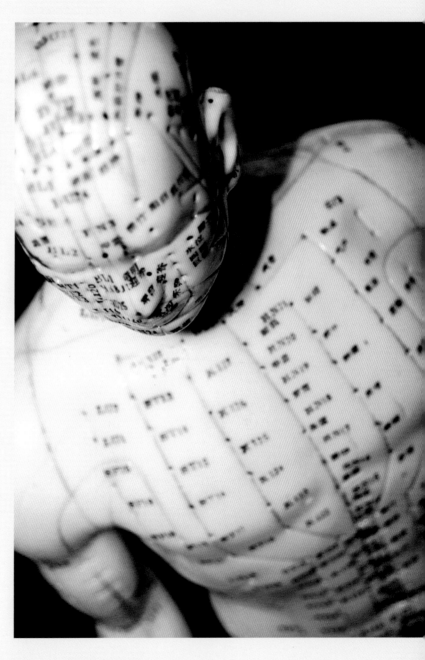

chi meridian massage

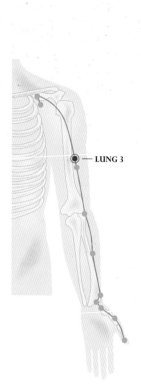

Massaging all your meridians in order, at one time, helps stimulate and circulate your chi throughout your body and normalize any excess or deficiency. One sample point is highlighted for each meridian for treating specific symptoms. After you have completed massaging the length of a meridian, go back and massage those points with your thumb or finger circling 36 times. As you will discover, one of the lovely aspects of the meridian system is that the points have very poetic names.

LUNG MERIDIAN MASSAGE
yin, metal

The lung meridian absorbs chi energy from the air you breathe. It controls respiration and oxygen content in your body, and has a close relationship with your heart and circulatory system. If you have nasal congestion, a cold, cough, asthma, skin problems or breathing problems, then massaging the lung meridian can help. If you are holding on to grief it will help you to release it. As you massage visualize your lungs in excellent health and your lung chi flowing in harmony. Let go of any grief or sadness you may be holding on to.

SELECTED POINT: Lung 3 'Celestial Storehouse'
For melancholy, depression, grief for loss of a loved one.

LARGE INTESTINE MERIDIAN MASSAGE
yang, metal

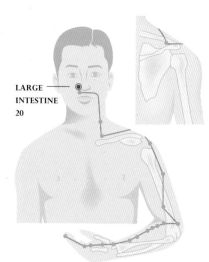

The large intestine meridian supports your body's ability to remove waste and absorb water. Massaging it will help sinus problems, nasal congestion, headaches, constipation, itchy skin, negative thinking, over-dependency, inability to release and move on, intestinal problems and a general lack of vitality. As you massage, visualize letting go of whatever you are holding on to that is preventing you from moving on.

SELECTED POINT: Large intestine 20 'Welcome Fragrance'
For releasing sinus or nasal congestion, and letting go of the past.

STOMACH MERIDIAN MASSAGE

yang, earth

The stomach meridian regulates the body's ability to take in food and fluid. Massaging this meridian helps with problems of self-nurturing, sugar addiction, over-working, overeating, cold sores, heavy legs, rough skin, hypertension, thinking too much and excessive worry. As you massage, visualize being able to eat a healthy diet consistently and to properly digest and make use of nutrients.

SELECTED POINT: Stomach 36 'Leg Three Miles' For extra energy to go the distance, strengthens defensive chi and relieves lower leg pain.

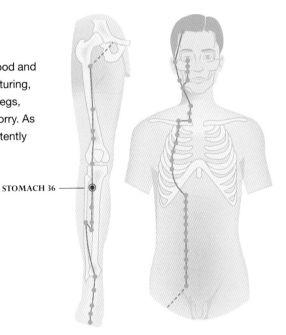

STOMACH 36

SPLEEN MERIDIAN MASSAGE

yin, earth

Your spleen meridian transforms food into energy, and regulates and maintains your body's blood supply. Massaging this meridian helps with problems of self-esteem and forgiveness, difficulties with self-care, isolation, overeating, obesity, nervous stomach, rounded back and heaviness in your legs. As you massage, imagine your spleen functioning properly. Generate compassion for yourself for any suffering that you may have endured. Commit to better self-care.

SELECTED POINT: Spleen 6 'Three Yin Intersection' For insomnia, menstrual cramps or PMS, male sexual issues and digestive disorders.

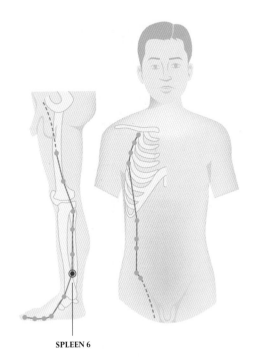

SPLEEN 6

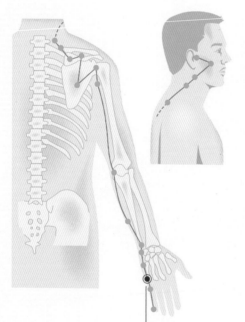

HEART 7

HEART MERIDIAN MASSAGE
yin, fire

Your heart meridian regulates your spirit, your body's blood and blood vessels, and the movement of your blood. Massaging your heart meridian helps with mental and physical fatigue, emotional distress, a weakened spirit, dizziness, palpitations, shortness of breath, lack of vitality, restlessness, absentmindedness, angina and heart organ problems. As you massage, visualize your heart as healthy. See it opening and your ability to love and receive love expanding.

SELECTED POINT: Heart 7 'Spirit Gate'
For emotional issues, anxiety, mania, insomnia, heart palpitations and angina.

SMALL INTESTINE 3

SMALL INTESTINE MERIDIAN MASSAGE
yang, fire

The small intestine meridian regulates the drawing out of nutrients and energy from your food. Massaging this meridian helps with issues of integrity and self-acceptance, deep emotional sadness, anaemia due to poor digestion, stiff neck, poor circulation in extremities, poor nutrient absorption and a tendency to overwork. As you massage, visualize your intestines as functioning in a healthy way. Feel any sadness fully and let it flow out of you.

SELECTED POINT: Small intestine 3 'Back Ravine'
For stiff neck, eye redness, inflammation and night sweats.

BLADDER MERIDIAN MASSAGE

yang, water

Your bladder meridian oversees your urinary organs and the excretion of urine. Massaging this meridian helps if you are easily frightened, find yourself constantly complaining, have difficulty with risk-taking and engaging in life, have frequent urination, bladder inflammation, tightness in back of legs, low back pain or sciatica. As you massage, visualize embracing life fully and fearlessly. Imagine that any urinary problems you have are cleared.

SELECTED POINT: Bladder 40 'Bend Middle'
For lower back pain, sciatica, summer heat and heat stroke.

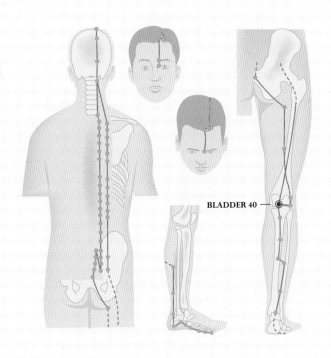

BLADDER 40

KIDNEY MERIDIAN MASSAGE

yin, water

Your kidney meridian oversees your reproductive energy, hormones and bones. Massaging this meridian can help with sexual and reproductive problems, osteoporosis, anxiety, fatigue, fear, pessimism, lack of determination, poor circulation in lower torso, impatience and restlessness. As you massage, become conscious of any habitual fear response and imagine relaxing and feeling safe in the moment. Visualize your kidneys full of energy and vitality.

SELECTED POINT: Kidney 27 'Shu Mansion'
For adrenal exhaustion, fatigue, immune deficiency, and opening and relaxing the chest.

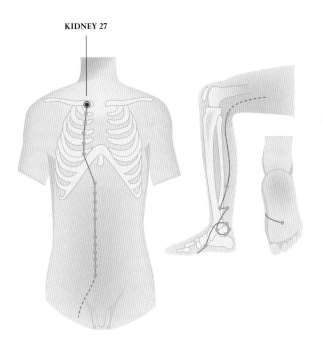

KIDNEY 27

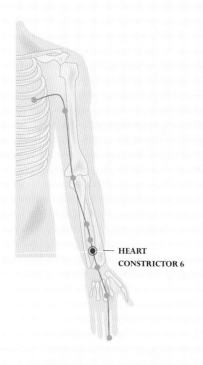

HEART CONSTRICTOR MERIDIAN
yin, fire

The heart constrictor meridian supports the heart meridian by overseeing, protecting and controlling circulation. Massaging your heart constrictor meridian helps with low blood pressure, palpitations, fatigue, insomnia, shortness of breath, restlessness and nervousness, memory problems, tingling in your fingers and chest pain. As you massage, visualize your heart functioning and blood flowing smoothly and efficiently. Imagine ways you can support your heart physically, emotionally and spiritually.

SELECTED POINT: Heart constrictor 6 'Inner Pass'
For nervousness, stress, memory problems and palpitations.

HEART
CONSTRICTOR 6

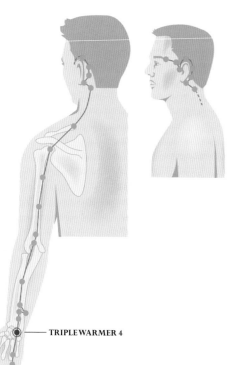

TRIPLE WARMER MERIDIAN MASSAGE
yang, fire

The triple warmer meridian circulates heat and balances water in three parts of your torso: the upper associated with respiration; the middle with digestion; and the lower with elimination. Massaging this meridian helps with obsessions, sensitivity to temperature changes, hydration, being overly cautious, lymphatic inflammations and tension in your arms. As you massage, imagine your body as warm and fully hydrated. Release any obsessive thoughts.

SELECTED POINT: Triple warmer 4 'Yang Pool'
For regulating temperature and water metabolism, dry mouth.

TRIPLE WARMER 4

GALL BLADDER MERIDIAN MASSAGE

yang, wood

Your gall bladder meridian regulates the creation of bile that aids in transforming your food into chi energy. Massaging your gall bladder meridian helps with difficulty making decisions, lack of creativity, lack of energy, obesity, insomnia, gallstones, bloating and migraines. As you massage, visualize being able to make decisions easily. Imagine relief from any problems with headaches.

SELECTED POINT: Gall bladder 8 'Name Valley Lead' For migraines with nausea/visual disturbance, and hangovers from alcohol or emotional upheaval.

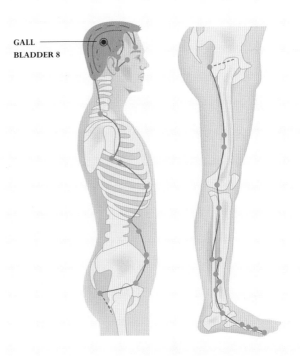

GALL BLADDER 8

LIVER MERIDIAN MASSAGE

yin, wood

Your liver meridian regulates the flow of chi throughout your body and maintains your body's blood supply. Massaging this meridian helps with problems of excessive anger, weak joints, lack of sexual energy, poor digestion, dizziness, stiff muscles, swollen stomach, and sugar, drug and alcohol addictions. As you massage, visualize any anger transforming into patience and tolerance. If you have problems with addiction admit to them and commit to getting help.

SELECTED POINT: Liver 3 'Great Surge' For all eye issues, chi and blood stagnation in the Middle Warmer, anger, irritability, insomnia, nausea and digestive problems.

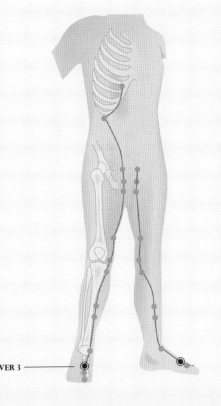

LIVER 3

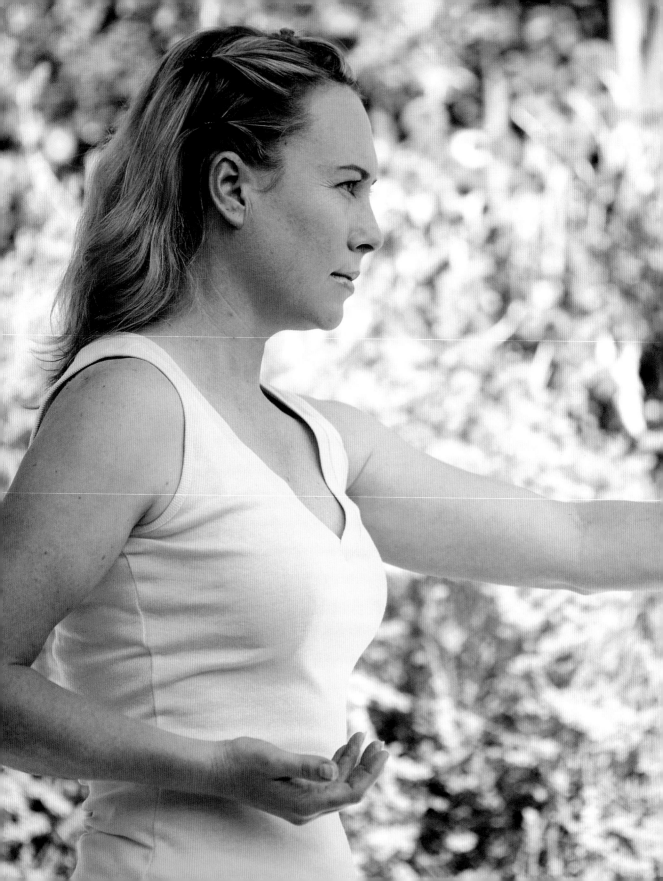

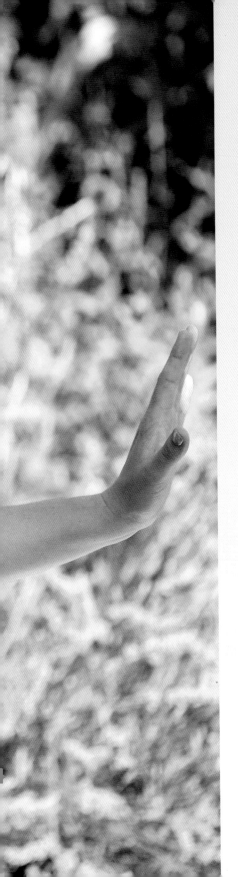

CHI AND DIET

The radiant face of a healthy person and the wholesome smell and flavour of a ripe peach reflect the chi that invigorates them. One of the ways you replenish chi is through the food you eat, therefore, from the Chinese perspective, what you eat is extremely important to maintaining your health and vitality. In the Western world, foods are evaluated for their protein, calorie, carbohydrate and vitamin/mineral content. In the Chinese and Taoist view, foods are considered according to their thermal energies, flavours and effects on specific organs and the body. In the Chinese approach to nutrition, no food is neutral and all foods are potentially medicine.

chi energy in food

Foods that have the most chi energy are fresh, locally grown, produced without chemicals or pesticides, and are whole and unrefined. Tired, limp, chemically laden vegetables will provide significantly less chi energy to your body than freshly picked organic ones. Studies have shown that organically grown foods have a higher nutrient content than those grown with pesticides in chemically fertilized soil.

The chi in animal foods suffers when cattle and hogs are confined and fed chemically laden grains instead of allowing them to roam and eat naturally. That they are often raised in inhumane conditions further compromises their chi, and that negative, diminished chi can be passed on to you. If you require animal protein in your diet, it is best to seek out organic, grass-fed animals that are humanely treated.

buying local

What does locally grown have to do with chi? Firstly, buying locally grown, organic food is good for your community; it is fresher, tastes better and is bursting with chi because it has had longer to ripen. Melons and tomatoes that have been allowed to grow on the vine until the last possible minute are mouth-wateringly fragrant and succulent, and bursting with nutrients and energy.

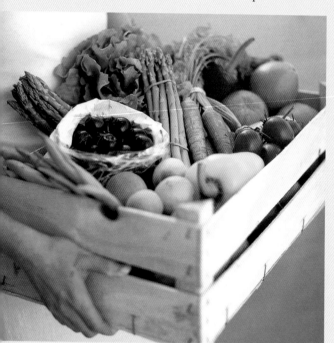

One of the best ways to replenish your chi is to eat plenty of fresh, organic vegetables.

Buying local foods keeps you in touch with the seasons and are the best foods for balancing your chi year round. Good, organic, local food also translates into more variety. When farmers are not producing standard fruits and vegetables to sell to supermarket chains, they will try out unusual varieties such as heirloom tomatoes or purple potatoes. When you eat locally grown organic food, you also absorb the positive chi energy of the farmer who is trying to grow foods in a way that truly nurtures and sustains the community.

whole versus refined foods

Chi is lost in food through the modern refining process that has been embraced by the food industry. Refined, denatured foods are lighter, sweeter, easier to chew and have longer shelf lives. Many of the products listed below not only have diminished chi, but are linked to many degenerative diseases such as diabetes and heart disease. Try to avoid:

- Refined grains such as white rice, white flour noodles and breads
- Refined oils and fat such as canola oil
- Partially hydrogenated fats such as margarine
- Refined white sugar or cane juice
- Highly processed low-fat dairy products.

Better choices are cooked wholegrains such as brown rice, chewy wholegrain breads and noodles made without added white flours, unrefined olive, sesame or flax oil, and whole, non-homogenized goat's milk, which is similar to human milk. Foods that are whole and unrefined, the way Mother Nature created them, have the most chi. If you are worried about full-fat dairy, it is better to eat very small amounts or none at all than to eat low-fat varieties. Our desire to overeat may in part be attributed to the missing chi and nutrients in the chemically laden, refined, denatured and genetically modified foods we eat. We unconsciously overeat in a futile attempt to absorb the chi that will never be there.

If possible, choose locally grown, organic vegetables for the best variety and quality.

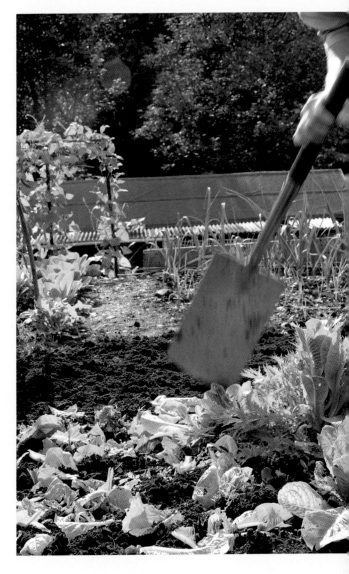

chi and food preparation

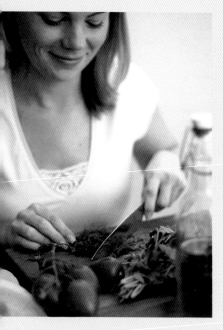

The manner in which you prepare your food has a profound effect on its chi.

Chi is not only taken in from food and air, it is transferred between people in interactions of all kinds. It is no surprise then, that the chi of the cook permeates the food. The way in which you prepare meals for yourself and others has a profound effect on the chi of the food. The quality, appearance, taste, balance and presentation of the food, and how you and others feel after eating, reflects the state of your chi physically, mentally, emotionally and spiritually.

maximizing chi in food

If, for example, you are resentful and angry while cooking, it will impart a feeling of anger into the food itself, which will diminish its chi. If you are worried about your budget and are selecting cheaper, poorer-quality foods or providing skimpy servings, you may impart a sense of deprivation, causing those you are feeding to binge later on junk food. Cooking in a rush in a chaotic kitchen can lend a feeling of anxiety to a meal, hardly a beneficial environment for ingesting nourishing chi. Whether cooking for yourself or others, here are a few suggestions for maximizing the chi in the food you serve.

- Be grateful that you have food to prepare.
- Express gratitude to the many people who were involved in growing or producing the food.
- Before you begin, make sure the kitchen is tidy and organized. Clean up as you go along and put everything not in use in its proper place.
- Honour the preparation and cooking of food and be pleased with your efforts, even if you are preparing something as simple as a nourishing bowl of porridge.
- Create a peaceful environment for preparing your food. Turn off the TV or CD player, and focus completely on what you are doing.
- Do not wear perfume or scent while preparing or cooking food as it will interfere with the smells of cooking.
- Set your intention to nurture and sustain yourself, family and friends in the best way you can.
- Start with the best-quality food you can find – fresh, whole, organic, unprocessed and bursting with chi energy.

- Study the healing powers of each food and try to prepare it simply without too many ingredients to bring out its full flavour and essence.
- Make an effort to set your table and present your food in an attractive, pleasing and harmonious way. Your table and food can be quite simple yet very appealing.

cooking methods

The method of cooking also affects the chi energy of food. Food cooked quickly without salt has a lighter feel. For a more harmonious, sweet and calming taste, cook on low heat for a longer period of time. Pressure cooking makes the chi in food more concentrated, hearty and strengthening. Steaming adds a moist yin quality, whereas baking is more yang and warming, and enhances sweet flavours.

As for cookware, stainless steel, clay, cast iron, glass and porcelain-coated or enamel-coated cast iron are recommended. Try not to use aluminium or non-stick coated cookware as it can interfere with the nutrition and chi energy of the food. If at all possible, avoid microwaves.

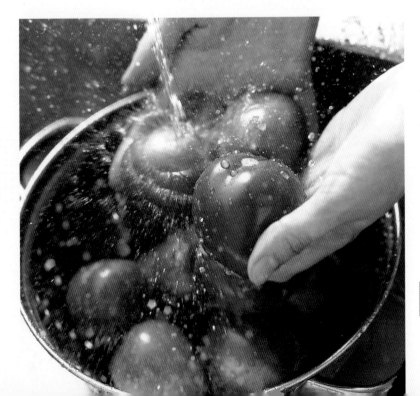

Stainless steel cookware is one of the best choices for preparing your food.

chi and raw food

Those who have embraced the raw food movement enthusiastically recommend that everyone eat a diet of raw fruits, vegetables, nuts and sprouted grains. The only cooking allowed is dehydration. The chi of raw food is certainly at its most pure and brimming with beneficial vitamins and enzymes. Think of a perfectly ripe peach just picked from the tree or a beautiful fresh raw vegetable salad. But raw food is not for everyone. The ability of individuals to assimilate food in a raw state will vary depending on the condition of their chi, and the state of their organ and meridian systems.

Raw foods are most beneficial for those who need a cleansing diet to counteract excess heat symptoms.

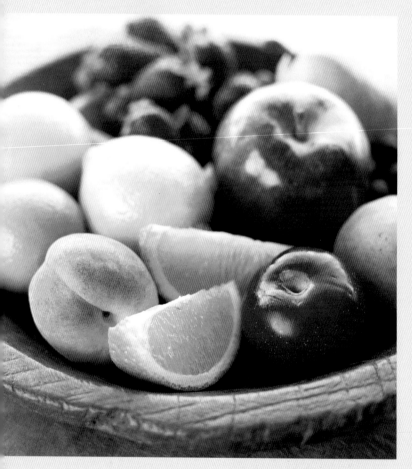

not for everyone

If you have what the Chinese call spleen chi deficiency or any cold condition, eating raw foods could damage your health by making your condition worse. If you have a cold condition and compromised metabolism, eating raw foods will rob your stomach area of the energy and heat it needs for digestion. This condition causes your body to have to work extra hard to digest food. And, because of your deficiency, raw food may pass through your system undigested, and its nutrients and chi will not be absorbed. With spleen chi deficiency, warm, slightly sweet, cooked foods are needed to restore health — brown rice, squash, oats, sweet potato, carrots and lamb. If you feel cold all the time, have a pale swollen tongue, feel weak and fatigued and have frequent urination, a raw food diet may not be for you.

On the other hand, if you have indulged in a rich diet of red meat, cheeses, alcohol, white flour pastas and desserts, you may end up with a damp condition combined with heat symptoms. Is your face or tongue red? Are you possessive and/or obsessed with someone? Are you overweight? Do you have slow digestion, anger and poor concentration? Then a period of cleansing with raw foods, combined with lighter cooked foods, is an excellent way to get your sluggish, stagnant liver chi moving again. Eating leafy green salads and raw vegetables would help clear your symptoms. There is no one way for everyone to eat.

ridding raw foods of parasites

Unfortunately, raw foods can have unwanted parasites and other micro-organisms. This is one reason why the ancient Chinese were not keen on raw foods. Parasites are not ancient history, and are very much with us today; even organic food can have parasites. But if you want to cleanse your system with the powerful chi of raw foods, there is a simple solution to these unwelcome guests. To remove parasites on the produce you plan to eat raw, soak it in a mild solution of one tablespoon of apple cider vinegar per gallon of water for 15 minutes.

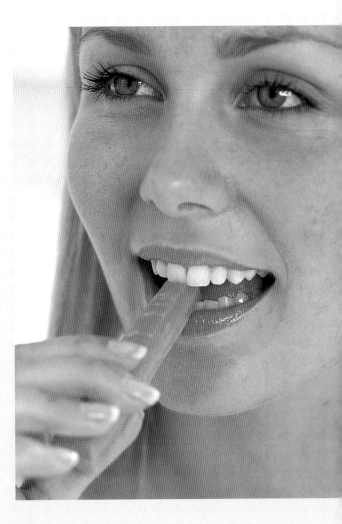

Soak raw foods in a mild solution of apple cider vinegar to rid them of any parasites.

yin and yang foods

Chi manifests in food as yin or yang – when thinking of yin and yang in relation to food, the words 'expansive' and 'contractive' are useful. Expansive foods are yin and contractive foods are yang. To stay in good health you need to balance your diet so that it does not become too yin (expanded, spacy and ungrounded) or too yang (tight, heavy and contracted).

determining yin/yang

Whether a food is yin or yang can sometimes be determined by its shape, weight, colour, water content, taste and region in which it is grown. Fruits and vegetables grown above ground are more expansive in shape and are usually yin, while those with a lengthened form, such as root vegetables, are yang. Heavier, denser foods like meat are more yang. Lighter foods like lettuce are yin. Foods that have colours in the cooler range, such as grapes, are more yin. Orange, red and brown foods, such as pumpkins are yang. Foods that are high in water content, such as melons, are more yin, while dry foods, such as grains, are more yang. Foods that are sweet and sour, like lemons and sugar, are more yin. Foods that are salty and bitter, like seaweed, are more yang. Foods that come from colder climates are more yang, while those from warmer, tropical areas tend to be yin.

Choosing the majority of your foods from the moderate category will help your chi energy stay balanced, healthy and flowing. However, the occasional indulgence in the extreme category is fine. The following chart will help you determine where your diet falls on the yin/yang spectrum.

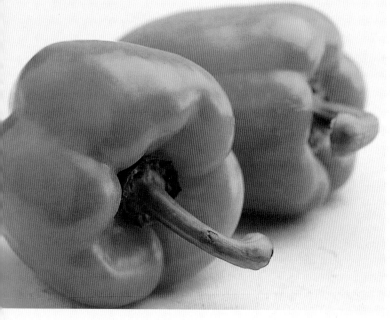

Peppers, no matter what colour, are part of the nightshade family and are considered yin.

Extreme yin and yang foods, and moderate foods

EXTREME YIN FOODS

Food group	Foods
Tropical fruits and nuts	Bananas, cashews, coconuts, figs, grapefruit, oranges, papayas, mangoes, lemons, tangerines, brazil nuts, hazelnuts, kiwi
Vegetables	White potato, tomato, peppers, aubergine
Processed grains	White and refined flours
Dairy	Butter, soft cheeses, cottage cheese, cream, ice cream, milk, yoghurt, frozen yoghurt, crème fraîche, sour cream
Oils	Olive, canola, corn, sesame, peanut
Other fats	Margarine, vegetable shortening, mayonnaise
Sweeteners	Corn syrup, honey, molasses, saccharine, white/brown sugar, fructose, maple syrup
Alcohol and beverages	Beer, wine, spirits, coffee
Additives and flavour-enhancers	Preservatives, chemical additives, spices

EXTREME YANG FOODS

Meats	Beef, bison, pork, lamb, veal, game meats
Poultry and poultry products	Chicken, duck, goose, ostrich, eggs
Dense, oily fish	Salmon, swordfish, tuna
Dairy	Hard cheeses
Additives and flavour-enhancers	Miso, soy sauce, tamari, salt

MODERATE FOODS

White meat fish/seafood	Clams, cod, flounder, haddock, halibut, scallops, shrimp, sole
Wholegrains	Brown rice, barley, buckwheat, corn, millet, oats, rye, wheat
Nuts and seeds	Almonds, hazelnuts, peanuts, pumpkin seeds, sunflower seeds, walnuts, pecans
Beans and bean products	Black, chickpea, kidney, lentils, lima, haricot, pinto, soy, split peas, tofu, tempeh, soy cheese
Sea vegetables	Dulse, arame, hijiki, Irish moss, kombu, nori, wakame
Root/stem vegetables	Carrots, cauliflower, radishes, parsnips, summer squash, turnips, winter squash, pumpkin, green beans, onion, burdock, sweet potato, yam
Green vegetables	Broccoli, Brussels sprouts, cabbage, celery, chives, spring greens, kale, cucumber, endive, lettuce, leeks, mustard greens, parsley, peas, spring onions, chard, watercress
Temperate fruits	Apples, pears, plums, apricots, blueberries, cantaloupe, cherries, grapes, peaches, raisins, raspberries, strawberries, watermelon
Sweeteners	Barley malt syrup, fruit juice, brown rice syrup

the five energies and flavours of food

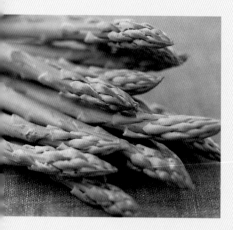

In the Chinese system, the thermal quality and flavour of food has an effect on your chi.

Not only can foods be assigned yin/yang or moderate qualities, they can also have particular energies with regard to their thermal nature, and can also be assigned one of five flavours.

the five energies

The five energies refer to the thermal nature of the chi energy in food — they could be 'cold', 'hot', 'warm', 'cool' and 'neutral'. But these labels do not refer to the actual temperature of the food as you eat it, but rather to the ultimate effect that it has on your body. You may be surprised to learn that tea has a cold energy, so even if you drink hot tea, it eventually will have a cold effect on your body. Coffee, on the other hand, is warming. Most meats are warming.

Knowing the thermal energy of foods is helpful for determining the best foods to eat for your body and condition. For example, if you have rheumatism, a cold condition, it is best to eat foods with a warm or hot energy that will relieve your pain. You should choose winter squash and forgo the watermelon. On the other hand, if you are experiencing a heat condition like skin eruptions, you may want to eat cooling foods such as barley or cucumber.

five energies and their foods

The following are some examples of foods in all five categories:
Cold Tea, watermelon, tomato, banana, seaweed
Cool Barley, lima beans, spinach, cucumber, strawberries, lettuce
Neutral Rice, aduki bean, beet, carrot, flax seed
Warm Parsley, parsnip, squash, almond
Hot Oats, black bean, cherry, walnut

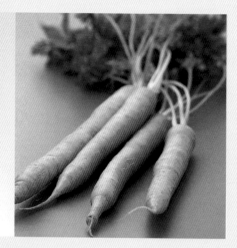

the five flavours

The five flavours of food are 'pungent', 'sweet', 'sour', 'bitter' and 'salty'. Not every food is a single flavour. Some foods, such as vinegar, are bitter and sour, and pork can be sweet and salty. Over many centuries, the Chinese have paid attention to the five flavours of foods and how they affect different yin and yang pairs of organs. For example, they discovered that pungent foods act on and help nourish the lungs and large intestine, and sour foods act on and help nourish the liver and gall bladder.

Locate a complete guide to the flavours of foods in a book on Chinese nutrition or on the Web, and begin to notice which flavours you tend to like and which you avoid. An ideal meal will have foods of each flavour in order to stimulate the chi in all organ systems. This is not hard to do. For example, using the foods below, prepare a lettuce salad with green onions and tomatoes, and a dressing made of olive oil, vinegar, a touch of honey and a dash of salt. Then have a handful of fresh cherries or a banana for dessert, and you will have a harmonious meal. In the following chapter we will explore in more detail the five energies and flavours, how they interact with the five elements and their related yin and yang organs.

five flavours and their foods

The following are some examples of foods in all five categories:
Pungent Spring onions, chives, clove, peppermint, ginger
Sweet Sugar, honey, coconut, cherry, pork, banana
Sour Lemon, pear, olive, plum, apple, grapefruit, tomato
Bitter Lettuce, asparagus, coffee, vinegar, wine
Salty Salt, barley, clam, crab, seaweed

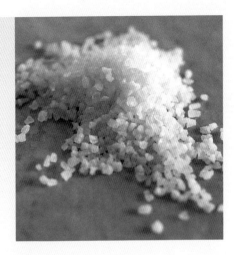

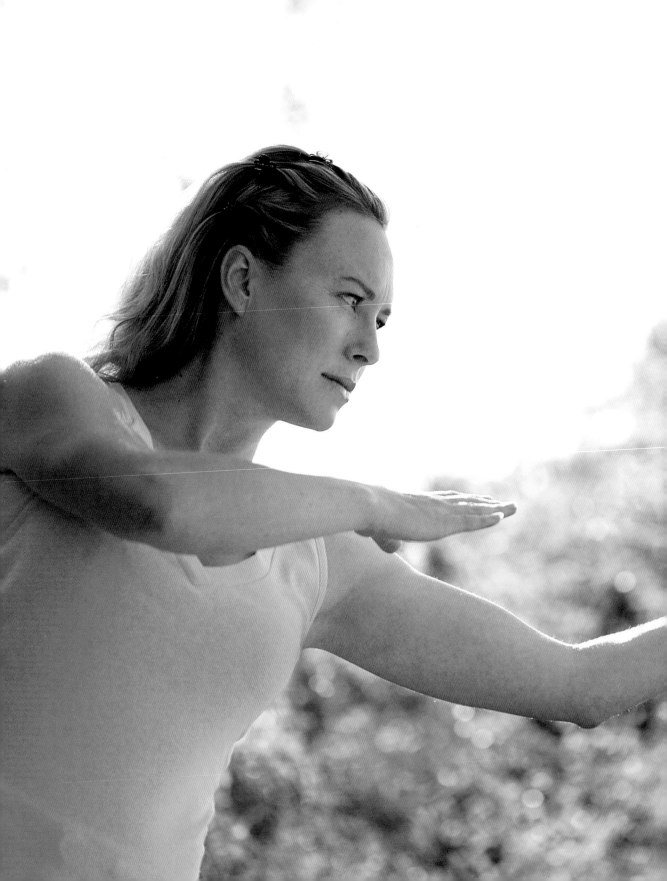

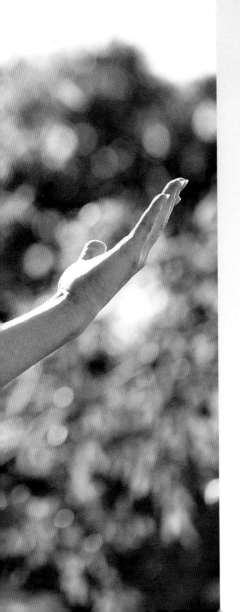

CHI, NUTRITION AND THE FIVE ELEMENTS

Earlier you were introduced to the concept of the five elements (see pages 38–47), and in this chapter we will further explore the elements as they relate to chi and nutrition. Although there are 12 meridians, the Chinese focus on ten internal organs for dietary treatment. These organs are considered in their yin/yang pairs and correspond to the five elements. To refresh your knowledge, go back to *Chi and the five elements* and review the element chart on page 41.

food as medicine

According to the Chinese, each food acts on or affects, one or more internal organs or elements. For example, if you eat celery, it acts on the stomach (the Earth element) and liver (the Wood element). The determination of the thermal nature, the flavours, the effects of various foods on the body, and which foods act on which organ or element, may, at first glance, seem arbitrary. But the Chinese have, over thousands of years, through observation and inductive and deductive methods, arrived at correspondences that have held up over time. Countless Chinese physicians throughout the ages have encouraged the healthy flow of chi by treating patients with dietary remedies using the Five Element System.

Eating according to the Five Element System can help balance your chi and maintain your health.

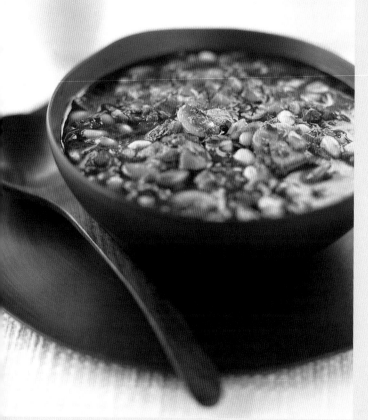

balancing the elements

In some cases, balancing the energy of one element requires attending to the nutrition of the organs in another. For example, you may have an imbalance in your Earth element because of problems with a deficient spleen. Simply eating earth-friendly plus spleen-strengthening foods and herbs can help. But, sometimes the reason your spleen or Earth element is weak or deficient is not because of something in your spleen, but because your liver or Wood element is congested and in a state of excess. In these cases just eating foods helpful to your spleen will be like continuously bailing a leaky rowboat. The 'leak' is being caused by your liver and Wood element that are too strong and invading your spleen. In this case, it is necessary to calm your liver with nourishing foods that are slightly bitter, such as asparagus, to bring the spleen into balance.

eat according to the seasons

The Chinese believe that the seasons have a profound effect on your health and well-being. Eating foods appropriate for the season is an important aspect of Chinese nutrition because your body adjusts when the seasons or climate changes. For example, if you live in a northern climate, your blood will begin to thicken in the autumn, a more yin time of year, as your body prepares for the cold winter months. You may unconsciously choose more concentrated foods, such as sourdough bread, cheese or olives. In the summer months, a more yang time of year, you may instinctively cook lighter fare – vegetables, salads and tofu. On a warm day, you may serve tortilla chips and salsas made with hot peppers. Hot peppers cause sweating, which has a cooling effect, providing a kind of natural air conditioning. Many of the hotter climates of the world – in Latin America, India and southern parts of Africa and China have hotter cuisines.

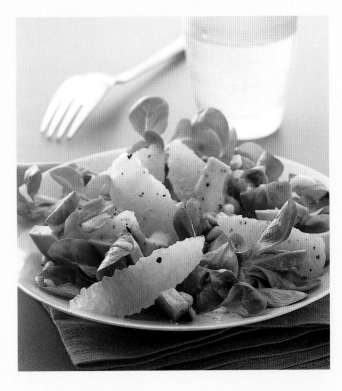

Lighter fare, such as a green salad, is an appropriate meal for the yang summer months.

The Taoist sages were highly attuned to nature. They believed that paying attention to the elements, the interaction of yin and yang and the cycling of the seasons is key to living a balanced life. Nurturing yang in the spring and summer, and yin in the autumn and winter through diet, exercise and meditation kept them in touch with the cycles of nature and their own bodies. In the rest of this chapter, we will explore nutrition as it relates to the five elements, their organs and the seasons associated with them.

nutrition and the Wood element

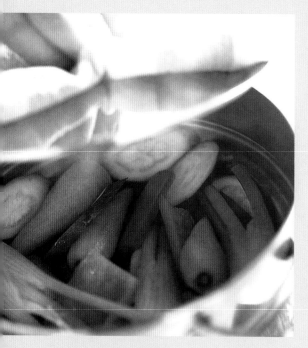

In the spring, emphasize lightly steamed vegetables and minimize the use of fats and oils.

Spring is the season of the Wood element, a time of growth and renewal, and for the Chinese, a perfect time to attend to the chi of liver and gall bladder. After a heavy winter diet of yang foods and fats, the liver and gall bladder need cleansing. This is a time when raw foods can be emphasized. Cooked foods should be lightly cooked or steamed, with minimal use of oil and fats.

liver and gall bladder

The liver and gall bladder are the most stressed, congested organs in the modern age. We take in too many fats, chemicals, preservatives, drugs — both prescribed and recreational — alcohol, environmental toxins of all kinds and refined denatured foods for these complex and delicate organs to handle. The result is often an overheated, stagnant and/or deficient liver and gall bladder chi. Our bodies rely on the liver and gall bladder for smooth-flowing chi throughout the body. If these are imbalanced, other organ systems will also be compromised as they are all interconnected. When the liver and gall bladder are healthy, we are relaxed, tolerant and patient. We are able to make decisions and be productive. When these organs are stressed, we have physical and emotional problems, including excess anger, depression, and thyroid and eye problems.

foods to balance liver and gall bladder chi

To bring a stagnant, swollen liver into harmony, start by eating less. Dramatically cut down on:
• Saturated fats found in red meat, cheese, and eggs
• Trans fats found in margarine and shortening
• Nuts
• Preservatives and chemical food additives
• Alcohol, processed and refined foods.

Begin to add foods that will help bring your liver out of its overheated, stagnant state:
- Pungent foods such as watercress, onion, turmeric, basil, ginger and horseradish, cauliflower, broccoli, Brussels sprouts
- Raw foods such as sprouts, fresh vegetables and fruits help cleanse the liver and restore chi flow
- Bitter and sour foods that reduce liver excess such as romaine lettuce, asparagus and chamomile tea
- All foods should be organic to avoid taxing the liver with pesticides and other chemical residues.

For restoring smooth flow of gall bladder chi, eat
- Unrefined grains, beans, vegetables and fruits
- Pears, parsnips, lemons, limes and turmeric help remove gallstones
- For several weeks, eat one or two radishes between meals and switch to flax oil on salads.

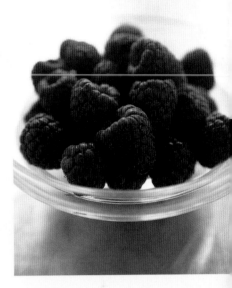

Temporarily eating raw fruits and vegetables can help restore a healthy flow of chi to a stagnant liver.

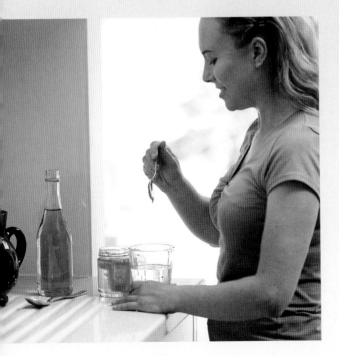

remedy for liver-related depression

Unless you are suffering from heat signs (red face, tongue, rashes), the detoxifying elements found in raw, unfiltered, organic apple cider vinegar will help cleanse and stimulate your tired liver out of stagnation. Constrained liver chi is considered one of the sources of depression by Chinese physicians.

1 Put two to three tablespoons of apple cider vinegar into a glass and dilute with water. You can add as much or as little water you prefer. Diluting with water is recommended so that the acids in the vinegar will not hurt your teeth.

2 Add raw, organic honey to the vinegar to help the digestion; it also contains beneficial vitamins and enzymes. Drink daily or until you feel some improvement in your mood.

nutrition and the Fire element

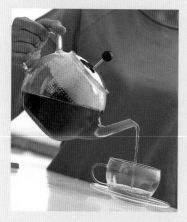

Drink herbal teas such as catnip and chamomile to calm the heart-mind of your Fire element.

Summer is the Fire element season, a time to get your creative juices flowing, to enjoy the fruits of your garden, and be expansive, joyful and relaxed. This is the time for brightly coloured fruits and vegetables to adorn your table. In the Chinese tradition, it is a good time to tend to the chi of your heart and small intestine. Fire is what keeps us warm, circulates our blood and helps us digest and assimilate food. Without good Fire chi, our health suffers.

heart and small intestine

The word for 'heart' in Chinese translates as 'heart-mind' and is thought to control blood circulation but also consciousness, spirit and the mind. The mind and emotions have a direct effect on the heart. Emotions cause chi circulation problems and feelings affect your heat rhythm. When you are afraid, your heart may pound in your chest and when you have angry thoughts, your pulse may race. Prolonged mental and emotional stress puts a strain on the heart and small intestine. When your heart is healthy, your blood flows smoothly. You have an open heart to people and experiences of all kinds. You have clarity of mind and emotion.

In Chinese medicine, the small intestine is thought to separate the pure from the impure. It sends nutrients to the spleen and waste to the large intestine. On a mental and emotional level, we need to separate out and absorb only the positive aspects and chi of our interactions with others, and eliminate any negative waste from our consciousness.

foods to balance and strengthen the heart and small intestine chi

One of the most important aspects of healing the Fire element is to calm the heart-mind. In our fast-paced lives we are guilty of mental hyperactivity, excessive thinking and worry, and excessive yang attitudes and behaviour. This stressful way of being has a negative effect on our mental, emotional and spiritual lives and therefore has a detrimental effect on the heart and small intestine. Foods that calm the mind and soul are good choices for balancing the chi of the Fire element. Try the following:

- Oyster shell in the form of calcium supplements are a good choice to help build the protective and nourishing yin of the heart
- Wholegrains of all sorts are calming and contain magnesium, which helps calcium absorption
- Cucumber, celery and lettuce also improve calcium absorption and strengthen heart tissue
- Chamomile, catnip, skullcap and valerian herbal teas will calm your nerves and help you sleep
- A small amount of goat's milk taken warm before bed is another way to help calm the heart-mind.

exploring healing mushrooms

Mushrooms of every variety are used in China for calming the nerves. Sixteenth-century Chinese medical texts say that the Reshi mushrooms mend the heart, and current research has found Reshi to be helpful in treating heart arrhythmias. Eating mushrooms often will boost your immune system, soothe your spirit and help strengthen and heal your Fire element chi.

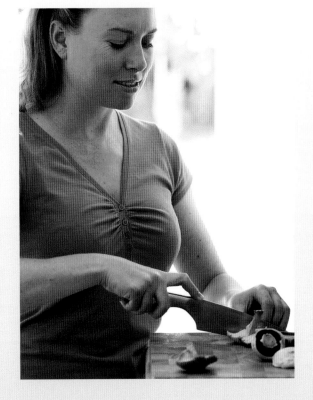

1 Investigate a good source of mushrooms, preferably organic. Look for morels, shiitake and maitake mushrooms, which were favourites of the ancient Chinese who used them to treat heart disease, and for promoting youthfulness and longevity. Today we know they can help lower cholesterol.

2 For one month, try a different organic mushroom with your meals each week, several times a week, either dried or fresh. Try creating mushroom sauces for meat, chicken or pasta. You can also find them as supplements available at health food stores.

nutrition and the Earth element

Late summer is the season of the Earth element, a time of transition between the yang of spring and summer and the coming yin of autumn and winter. This is a time of your centre – your spleen/pancreas and stomach – and a time to work on centring physically, emotionally and spiritually. It is a time for reflection on the cycles of nature and the earth.

spleen/pancreas and stomach

By looking after your Earth element you will help maintain a healthy weight.

The Earth element's organs, the spleen/pancreas (pancreas in modern physiology) and the stomach, are responsible for the digestion and distribution of food and nutrients. Chi energy generated from your food gives you warmth and vitality, healthy tissues and optimal brain function. If your spleen/pancreas and stomach are healthy, you will have good digestion and be able to nurture yourself and others easily. You will have a strong body and will be experienced by others as emotionally responsible and stable. If your Earth element is compromised, you will feel tired and stuck in a cycle of compulsive behaviours. You may be overweight and have elevated blood sugar.

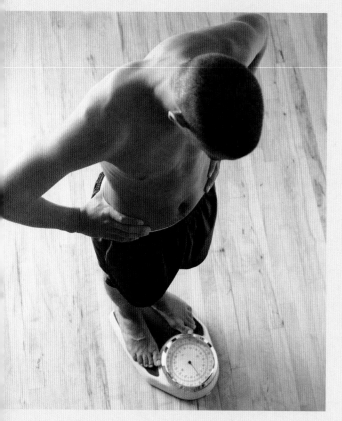

foods to balance and strengthen the spleen/pancreas and stomach chi

There are two main disturbances of spleen/pancreas chi that require slightly different foods to heal, although they often manifest simultaneously. The first is weak spleen/pancreas chi caused by being malnourished from eating overly processed, denatured foods; and the second is having an excess of dampness or mucus in the body, caused by overeating, late night eating and too much meat, dairy, sweets, ice cream and fats. There may also be underlying emotional reasons for the imbalances.

healing weak spleen/pancreas

Weak spleen/pancreas chi manifests as nervous indigestion, anaemia, chronic diarrhoea and pain in the abdomen. To heal weak or deficient spleen/pancreas chi, eat foods that are neutral or warming.

- Avoid raw or cooling foods as they can cause further harm. Try cooked grains, such as brown rice, oats or spelt, and vegetables that have a sweet or pungent flavour such as winter squash, carrots, parsnips, turnips, sweet potato, chickpeas and black beans.
- To these you can add onions, leeks, ginger, garlic, black pepper, cinnamon and nutmeg.
- Small amounts of chicken, beef or lamb in a soup can be helpful.

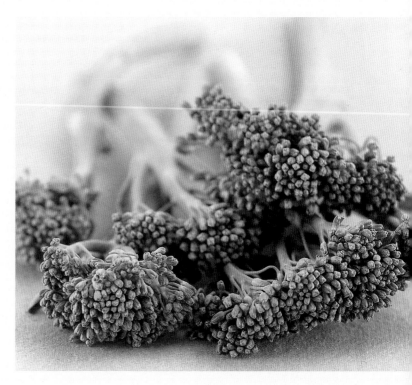

Heal your Earth element with simple meals of lightly cooked, organic vegetables.

healing damp spleen/pancreas

Dampness is an overly moist condition in the body and manifests as swelling, yeast infections, cysts, tumours and cancers. Dampness can invade any part of the body including the heart and lungs. If you have dampness affecting your spleen/pancreas and stomach, you may have a bloated abdomen and watery stools. You may have a heavy feeling in your body and/or numbness and have difficulty moving. The best approach to healing dampness is to:

- Eat fewer animal products
- Avoid refined over-processed foods, and foods high in fat and mucus-forming such as ice cream and dairy products
- Eat simple cooked meals made up mostly of vegetable foods
- Eat foods that have a drying effect such as rye, corn, aduki beans, celery, lettuce, green onions and chamomile tea
- Small amounts of raw, organic honey can be used
- If you crave dairy, raw goat's milk or yoghurt has an astringent quality and will not cause dampness in the body
- Address any emotional reasons for overeating or eating poorly such as anger or depression.

nutrition and the Metal element

Autumn is the Metal element's season, a time of shifting physically and psychologically from the yang of spring and summer to the yin of autumn and winter. This is the time of harvest, of gathering food and a time for gathering your thoughts. Metal is about organization and mental focus. You become more aware of the aroma of food baking in the oven. The aromas are received through your sense of smell, which is governed by the Metal element and the lungs. The foods should be more concentrated to prepare the body for the coming cold months. Baked wholegrain breads and root vegetables are great in the autumn.

Autumn, the season of the Metal element, is a perfect time to enjoy wholegrain breads.

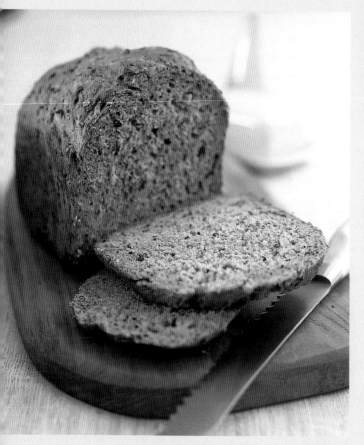

lungs and large intestine

The lungs take in chi from the air and it is mixed with the chi gathered from food. Lung chi helps protect the surface of the body and the mucous membranes from bacteria and viruses. When your lung chi is healthy and strong you will have a good immune system, and be able to be organized and effective. You will know when to hold on and when to let go in business, relationships and with your possessions. The large intestine releases the parts of food that are waste and no longer needed, but if your large intestine chi is weak or compromised, you may find yourself having unhealthy attachments to people and things that are not beneficial.

foods to balance and strengthen lung and large intestine chi

Pungent foods are at the top of the list for cleansing and protecting the lungs and large intestine chi.

Try the following foods:
- Hot peppers and chillies
- White pungent foods like onion, garlic, turnips, horseradish, daikon and white pepper
- Mucilaginous foods such as seaweeds, flaxseeds and fenugreek are good for the mucous membranes
- Foods with lots of beta-carotene like carrots, watercress, squash and mustard greens renew the membranes of the lungs and large intestine
- Green foods with chlorophyll, such as wheat or barley grass and blue-green algae help cleanse the lungs from the ravages of air pollution and toxic fumes
- Increased fibre intake, the indigestible parts of wholegrains, fruits and vegetables, is essential for healthy lung and large intestine chi. For lung and large intestine health, and especially for lung and colon cancer prevention, start by increasing your fibre intake by at least 30 per cent, and perhaps more over time.

deep breathing

Grief is the emotion associated with the Metal element. Repressed grief and sadness causes long-term damage to the lungs and large intestine. Since emotional repression causes shallow breathing, deep breathing is a way to start. If any sadness or grief arises, do not repress it but let it come out. Food remedies and nutritional support for your Metal element will not be as effective until your grief is resolved.

1 Set aside quiet time each day to simply relax for five minutes and breathe.

2 Breathe in deeply through your nose, all the way down to your abdomen, so that you feel the sides of your ribs expand. Do this to the count of five. Hold for a count of two, then exhale through your mouth to the count of five.

3 Repeat for a few minutes each day.

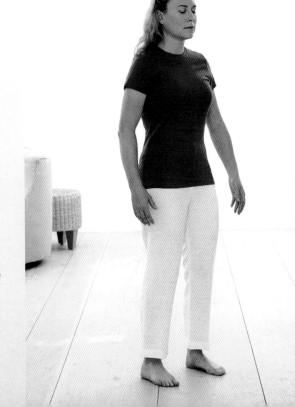

nutrition and the Water element

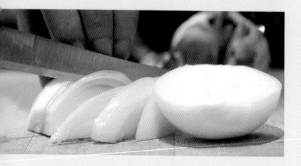

Winter is the season of the Water element. It is the most yin time of year, a time to be introspective, meditate and receptive to any spiritual realizations that may emerge. For both men and women, it is a time to embrace the yin – the receptive, yielding, feminine aspects of our personality. We also may appear softer and rounder, having put on a few pounds, a natural tendency to store chi energy during the winter months.

Warming foods like onions and garlic can help to heal kidney yang deficiency, a cause of sexual dysfunction.

kidneys and the bladder

The Water element organs are the kidneys and bladder. In the Western view these organs are primarily related to the production of urine. But in the Chinese view, besides governing urine production and water metabolism, these organs include the function of the adrenals and the sexual/reproductive organs. They are also associated with the bones, teeth and hearing. Your kidney chi energy has a lot to do with longevity and vitality in old age. If your Water element chi is healthy you will feel relatively safe and secure in the world. Others will notice your calm demeanour and ability to work without stress. If not, you may be fearful, have phobias and be easily startled. You may be agitated, nervous and insecure and not very dependable.

foods to balance and strengthen kidney and bladder chi

The pleasing sounds of cooking coming from the kitchen are now more important than the aromas. Both salty and bitter foods are appropriate and appealing during the winter as they help bring warmth to the core of the body.

healing kidney yin deficiency

If you have dizziness, ringing in your ears, a fast pulse, red tongue and dry mouth and nocturnal emissions, and if you are agitated and nervous you

may have kidney yin deficiency. Foods that nurture the kidney yin include:
- Barley, tofu, beans, melons, blueberries, water chestnuts, wheat germ, seaweeds, green beans and black sesame seeds
- Small amounts of crab, clams, eggs and pork
- Avoid warming foods such as coffee, alcohol, tobacco, lamb, cinnamon, ginger and hot spices
- Avoid overeating.

healing kidney yang deficiency

If you have kidney yang deficiency, you may feel cold, have a pale complexion, and weak knees and lower back. Other symptoms are lack of sexual desire, frequent urination and an enlarged pale tongue. You may be lethargic and unproductive. Because the yang warming function of your kidneys is not working, choose warming foods such as:
- Walnuts, onions, garlic, leeks, quinoa
- Chicken, lamb and trout
- Warming spices such as cinnamon, black pepper, and ginger are fine.

healing damp heat in the bladder

Bladder infections are a sign of damp heat in the bladder. Symptoms are burning, painful urination, fever and cloudy urine. The majority of your foods should be chosen to remove dampness and heat. Foods that are bitter and cooling are the best choices. Eat lightly and make soups from any of the following ingredients:
- Aduki bean, lima beans, celery, potatoes with skins, asparagus, mushrooms
- Drinking diluted unsweetened cranberry juice and dandelion tea is also helpful.

Finally, to keep your Water element chi balanced and flowing, stay hydrated with plenty of pure, filtered water.

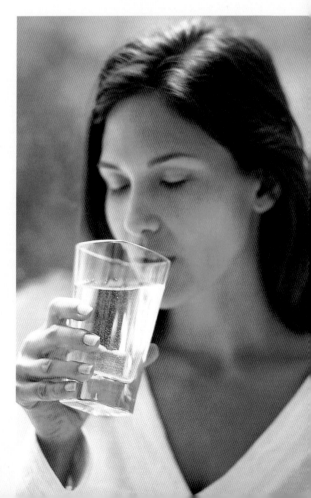

It is important to nourish your Water element with plenty of pure filtered water.

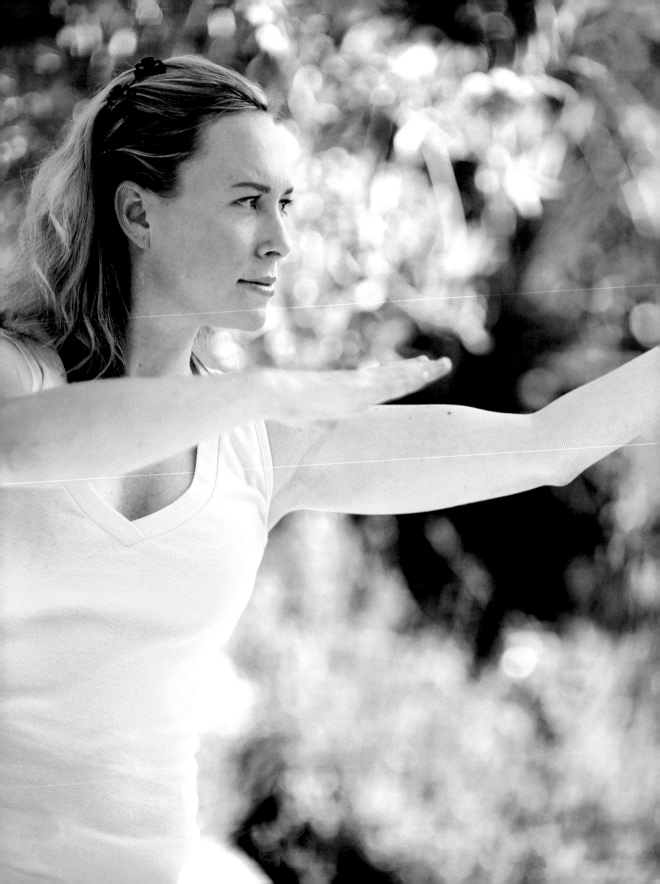

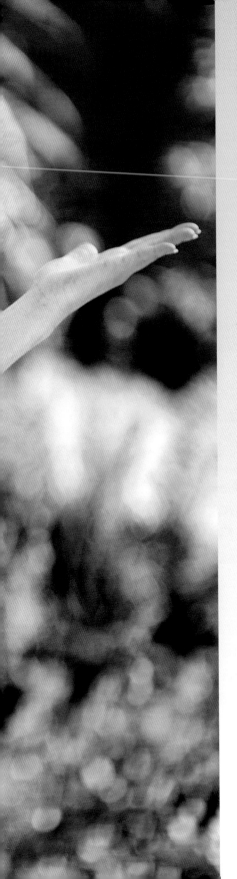

CHI AND
EXERCISE

All exercise encourages the flow of chi in the body, including a traditional workout at the gym, dance or aerobics. The Taoist approach to exercise is internal, preferring to move energy rather than muscle. Emphasis is put on the circulation of blood and chi and the internal massaging of organs and meridians. Fitness is achieved from the inside out. The Taoist practices of Chi Kung and T'ai Chi are excellent alternatives to Western exercise for promoting health, vitality and cardiovascular fitness.

chi and relaxation

Chronic tension in the body inhibits the flow of chi. Before you can benefit from other chi-enhancing exercises in this chapter, it is helpful to address the overall chronic tension you may be carrying in your body. Your body contains the imprints of your emotions – grief, anger and sadness come and go, but their residue can stay stored in your cells for a lifetime.

Hunched shoulders might tell of a sense of childhood shame and low self-esteem, a holding of tension in the pelvic area may be from psychological and emotional conflicts about sex, or even from past sexual abuse. You may have a clenched jaw from chronic anger and find yourself grinding your teeth at night. Tension can be held in any part of your body, even in your scalp.

The manner in which you focus your mind on a daily basis also can contribute to stress and chronic tension. A perpetual narrow mental focus on tasks at work, on a TV or computer screen, and on excessive and repetitive rumination about worries and problems can cause untold damage to your body and mind. It is as if your mind is stuck in third gear and is incapable of trying out other, more spacious and relaxing ways of being in the world.

The problem is that this held tension is so habitual and feels so natural, that you may not even be aware of how it contorts your body and mind, or the toll it is taking on your health. Before beginning any of the chi exercises it is useful to practise the following relaxation exercise.

body scan for releasing chronic tension

1 Lie on the floor with your legs stretched out, feet slightly wider than your hips. Place your arms at about 45 degrees to your body with your palms facing upwards, hands and fingers relaxed.

2 Flex your right ankle, then tense your foot, your calf muscle, your knee and slightly contract your thigh muscle. Now tighten your whole right leg. Hold, then breathe out and release, letting all the tension flow out through your foot. Repeat with your left leg.

3 Squeeze your buttocks one at a time and then together as tightly as you can. Release and feel the tension flowing away.

4 Focus on your lower and upper abdominal muscles, draw your navel back towards your spine as far as you can, then breath out and release, allowing all the tension to drop away.

5 Bring your awareness to your back muscles. Tense your back muscles. As you breathe out, let your muscles sink down into the floor.

6 Contract your chest muscles as tightly as you can, then release, breathing out any tension.

7 Bring your awareness to your shoulders. Tighten your right shoulder muscle, then release, letting the shoulder sink into the floor. Do the same with your left shoulder.

8 Tense your right arm muscles and squeeze your hand and fingers as tightly as you can, lifting your arm slightly off the floor. Release and feel the tension flowing down and out your fingertips. Do the same with your left arm.

9 Tense the muscles of your neck and throat. Clench your jaw tightly and scrunch up your whole face, then release.

10 Breathe into your lower abdomen and hold your breath for a few seconds, then release. Breathe and hold three times. Then rest and feel how your body feels without tension.

11 When you are ready, stand up and notice how your body feels when relaxed.

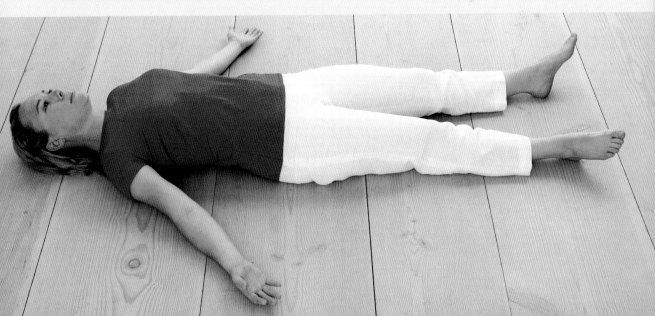

meridian stretches

The following six exercises are simple and quick stretches that have been designed to stimulate and balance the chi in your 12 meridians. All six stretches can be completed in five minutes.

lung and large intestine meridian stretch

1 Stand with your feet slightly more than shoulder-width apart. Put your hands behind your back with your palms facing backwards and hold them together by hooking your thumbs together.

2 Keeping your knees straight, bend forwards as you exhale. Stretch your arms overhead as far as they will go, then quietly begin to inhale and exhale. Do not force the stretch, but relax into it. Notice any sensations along the lung and large intestine meridians in your arms. Inhale and exhale three times and release.

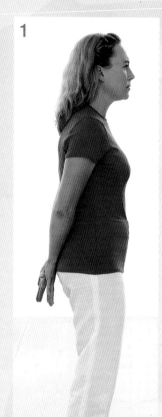

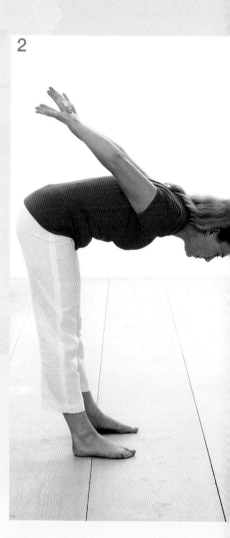

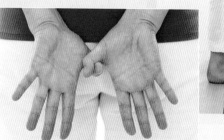

kidney and bladder meridian stretch

1 Sit on the floor with your legs stretched out in front of you. Keep your heels together and your toes apart.

2 Keeping your knees straight, exhale as you bend forwards to reach for your toes. Face your palms outwards. Stretch as far as you can and take a deep breath. The tension you feel along your back and the backs of your legs down to your feet are your kidney and bladder meridians. Exhale. Inhale and exhale three times and release.

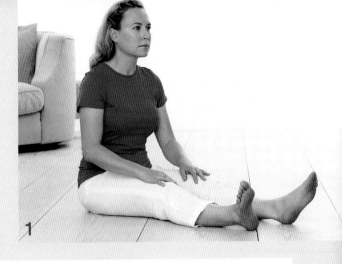

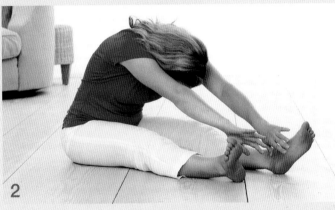

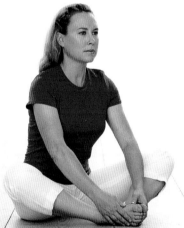

heart and small intestine stretch

1 Sit on the floor. Place the soles of your feet together in front of you by bending the knees out to the sides. Pull your feet in towards you by grasping your toes.

2 Bend forwards while exhaling and stop when you have stretched to your limit. Breathe in to fill up with chi. The lines of tension you feel in your arms are your heart and small intestine meridians. Inhale and exhale three times and release.

stomach and spleen meridian stretch

1 Sit on the floor in a kneeling position.

2 Slowly lean backwards. As you lean back, slowly move your feet out from under your bottom so it rests on the floor.

3 Keep going until your shoulders and upper back are also resting on the floor and extend your arms over your head. Breathe in and stretch your whole body. The lines of tension you feel down the front of your body and legs are the spleen and stomach meridians. Inhale and exhale three times and release.

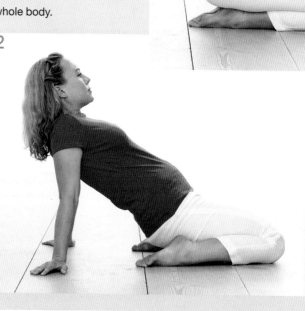

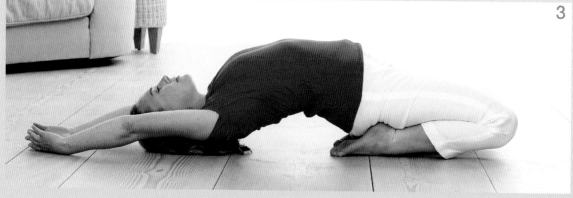

heart constrictor and triple warmer meridian stretch

1 Sit cross-legged on the floor. Cross your arms one over the other and grab the opposite knees.

2 Exhale, bending forwards as far as possible using your arms to pull your upper body down to the floor. Let your head hang down. Take a deep breath. The lines of tension on the outside and inside of your arms are the heart constrictor and triple warmer meridians. Release and feel the meridians relax. Repeat three times.

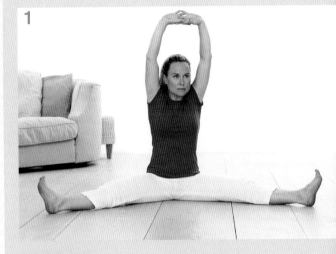

1

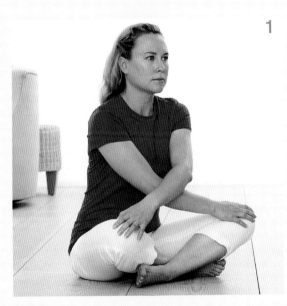

1

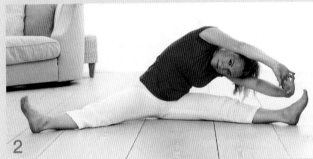

2

liver and gall bladder meridian stretch

1 Sit on the floor with legs spread as far apart as you can. Keep your knees straight. Clasp your hands high over your head and turn your palms upwards.

2 Keep facing forwards as you exhale and bend down to one side. Inhale deeply. The lines of tension along the outside and inside of your legs are the liver and gall bladder meridians. Inhale and exhale three times on each side.

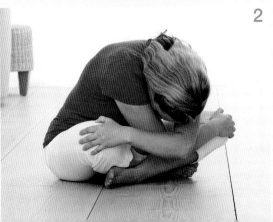

2

exercise East and West

Exercise and an active lifestyle have many health-related benefits. A lack of exercise is detrimental to overall health and is associated with an assortment of serious health problems. A sedentary lifestyle has been linked to cancer, cardiovascular disease, hypertension and diabetes. Our bodies were designed to move – to walk, to dance, to run – and we have a skeleton, muscles, ligaments and tendons that make all sorts of movements possible.

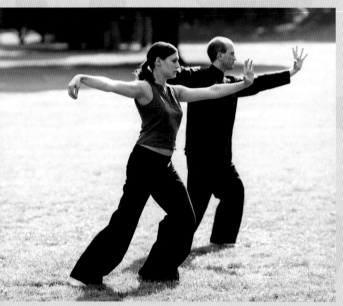

T'ai Chi is one of the best exercises for maintaining health and can be practised well into old age.

sedentary modern life

Our modern lifestyles keep us in an unnatural, almost motionless state for much of the day. We know this is not a good situation, yet we find ourselves just too tired to exercise after work. Low energy could be attributed to a lack of muscle tone and aerobic capacity, but the real culprit may be that our chi circulation is constrained, sluggish and even stagnant from lack of movement. Our breathing may be shallow further depressing our chi. The end result is that our overall health suffers because our organ systems are not being nourished by the chi they need to function properly. We put ourselves at risk of more serious illness and disease.

ancient Chinese exercise regimes

Most traditional exercise, such as walking, aerobics or weightlifting, will encourage chi to move, but the best exercises for moving chi are the ancient Chinese Taoist practice of Chi Kung and the internal martial art T'ai Chi. Thousands of years ago, Taoist sages realized that inactivity was a major cause of illness. Being greatly interested in longevity, they developed Chi Kung exercises for circulating chi and preventing and curing disease. Later, the internal martial arts were developed, which, in addition to providing self-defence, have similar positive effects on health and chi circulation. Today, in China and around the world, Chi Kung and T'ai Chi are practised to promote health and well-being.

long-term benefits

Not only do Chi Kung and T'ai Chi circulate chi, but these gentle exercises can provide many of the same benefits as working out at the gym without the dangers of joint injury or exhaustion from over-exercising. High-impact aerobics can produce health benefits over the short term, but the long-term implications of such exercises are questionable. Over time, they can cause damage to the joints and internal organs. Exercises such as running and jogging, when practised to excess, can sometimes injure the heart rather than strengthen it.

Because they are made up of slow-moving or even stationary exercises, it may seem that Chi Kung and T'ai Chi do not provide the same degree of cardiovascular fitness as high-impact exercises, such as jogging or aerobic dancing. However, this is not true. When the movements of Chi Kung or T'ai Chi are performed quickly or in a lower stance, they can have the same beneficial effect on the cardiovascular system as high-impact exercises, but without the stress and strain.

T'ai Chi and Chi Kung can provide many of the same benefits as working out at the gym.

Some medical experts warn that ongoing strenuous exercise, rather than being beneficial, may actually shorten your life. Instead, they recommend exercises that are gentler on the body, yet still provide movement of the legs, torso and arms, improve flexibility and strength, and build aerobic capacity. These exercises need to be effective in preventing obesity but not be so exhausting as to deplete the body, and, ideally, they should be suitable for all ages and body types. Chi Kung and T'ai Chi fit all of these requirements. Not only do they provide excellent physical exercise, they also lend themselves to meditation and provide an opportunity to relax the mind.

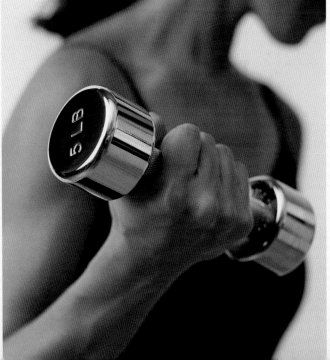

what is chi kung?

Chi Kung is an aspect of Chinese medicine that combines movement, meditation and regulation of breathing to enhance the flow of chi. The words Chi Kung mean 'energy cultivation'. Chi Kung is a health practice with strong meditative and metaphysical aspects designed to help nourish and circulate chi. It enhances ancestral chi and helps you access and make use of the chi energy of the universe.

integrating body, mind and spirit

Chi Kung works directly with chi energy for the purpose of integrating body, mind and spirit. Some exercises help you increase your store of chi, while others help you to move and circulate it by using your mind and meditative techniques. Practising Chi Kung on a regular basis can help you prevent and heal illnesses and develop a spiritual relationship with nature and the universe. With advanced practice you can learn to transfer your chi to others and help them replenish depleted energy.

The slow and gentle movements of Chi Kung encourage the circulation of chi throughout the entire meridian system.

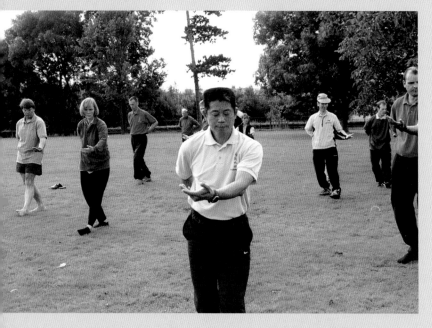

China has a long history of developing exercises designed to enhance chi movement in the body. In the third century BCE, a physician named Hua-t'uo created a health practice called the Movement of the Five Animals, which consisted of imitating the movements of the tiger, deer, bear, ape and bird. He believed that the body needed exercise to help with digestion and circulation, and that only by exercising could one live a long and healthy life. His exercises, probably the earliest precursor of Chi Kung and T'ai Chi, are still taught in China and around the world.

Indian Buddhist influences

Later, in the sixth century CE, Indian Buddhist meditation master Bodihdharma came to the Shaolin Monastery in China, and saw that the monks were in poor physical condition from too much meditation and not enough movement. He created the Eighteen Hands of the Lohan Chi Kung exercises. The movement of chi energy through the practice of these exercises opened the energy channels of the body and facilitated meditative realizations.

Many versions of Chi Kung exercises were developed, refined and passed down over the centuries from teacher to disciple as closely guarded secrets. Once shrouded in secrecy, Chi Kung practices are widely available to anyone who wants to learn. Today, millions of people in China and around the world regularly practise Chi Kung to maintain health.

the benefits of practising chi kung

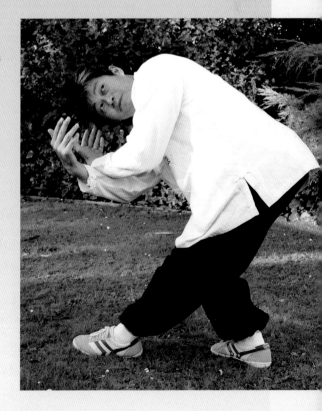

- Strengthens, balances and nourishes all your meridians and organ systems, which helps to prevent illness.
- Loosens tight muscles. Instead of building strength through muscle contraction, Chi Kung builds stronger muscles by loosening them and letting the chi flow through.
- Improves heart and lung function through slow, deep breathing. Conscious deep breathing combined with energy movement provides more oxygen to the cells than regular aerobic activity.
- Strengthens the nervous system, improves motor coordination, relieves stress.
- Improves circulation and vascular function.
- Can be practised by the physically weak and ill.
- Improves balance.
- Increases flexibility in the ligaments.
- Speeds recovery time from operations.
- Balances the emotions.
- Promotes the opening of energy channels for spiritual realizations.

what is t'ai chi?

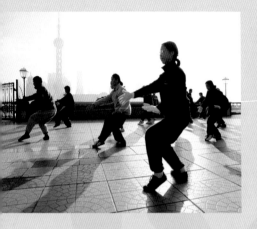

The term 'T'ai Chi Chuan' means 'Supreme Ultimate Force'. This notion refers to the Chinese concept of yin and yang, the idea of a dynamic duality that pervades all things. The practice of T'ai Chi Chuan or T'ai Chi consists of learning a sequence of movements called a form. These movements, originally martial in nature, are kicks, punches, strikes and blocks. However, in T'ai Chi these movements are performed in graceful, slow motion with smooth, seamless transitions. For most practitioners today, the focus is not on martial applications but on health and longevity. As in Chi Kung, T'ai Chi encourages the circulation of chi within the body, thus enhancing health and vitality.

T'ai Chi is practised by millions of people around the world every day.

Taoist roots

Although T'ai Chi was developed as a martial art, the roots of T'ai Chi rest in Taoist philosophy. The Taoist monk Chang San-Feng, who lived in the 14th century CE, is considered the father of T'ai Chi Chuan. After much observation, Chang concluded that most martial forms were too vigorous, too violent and relied too heavily on physical strength. He set about creating a new meditative martial art that relied on internal chi power and the Taoist belief that yielding overcomes aggression and softness overpowers hardness. He created the fundamental Thirteen Postures of T'ai Chi. These postures corresponded to the eight basic trigrams of I Ching, a Chinese system of divination, and the Five Element System of Chinese medicine.

t'ai chi today

Today, there are many schools of T'ai Chi in China and around the world, and the forms have grown from 13 to hundreds of movements. Yang, Wu and Chen are the most well-known styles – all named after the families who created them. Of these, the Yang style is the most popular. The Simplified Yang Style Form is the easiest form of T'ai Chi to learn and the most accessible to people of all ages and physical abilities.

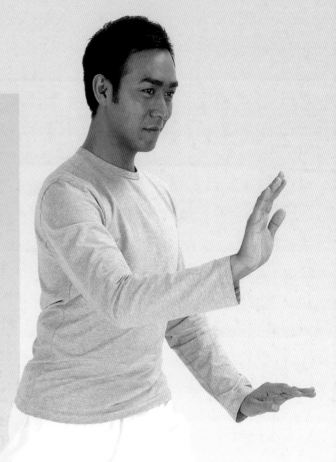

the benefits of practising t'ai chi

- Provides the movement the sedentary body needs.
- Massages the meridians and internal organs.
- Stretches muscles and ligaments.
- Promotes the flow of blood, lymph, joint, brain and spinal fluids.
- Increases chi flow and helps to store chi.
- Improves balance, body posture and alignment.
- Increases aerobic capacity.
- Improves muscle strength.
- Increases range of motion in the joints.
- Strengthens the legs.
- Alleviates chronic pain.
- Improves sexual stamina and response.
- Enhances brain function.
- Reduces stress; promotes emotional and mental relaxation.
- Promotes longevity.
- Improves sleep.
- Lowers and regulates blood pressure.
- Suitable for people of any age or physical or mental capability.
- Promotes a peaceful and quiet mind.

the three corrections

There are three important adjustments or corrections to make when you practise Chi Kung or T'ai Chi. They are the corrections of posture, breath and mind. Before beginning any chi exercise, first practise the body scan relaxation technique (see pages 86–87), then bring the following adjustments to mind, and try to remain conscious of them throughout your practice. You may find them applicable for accomplishing anything in life.

correction of body posture and movement

Each posture or movement in Chi Kung or T'ai Chi will have its own unique form, but the following general guidelines apply to all chi exercises:

1 Imagine your head is suspended from above by a thread. This keeps your posture in alignment but not rigid and energizes your body. Keep your mouth closed with tongue touching the roof of your mouth behind your front teeth. This completes a circuit for chi.

2 Relax your shoulders downwards and keep them slightly rounded to open your shoulder, elbow and wrist joints and to facilitate abdominal breathing. Relax your chest inwards so that it becomes slightly hollow to facilitate abdominal breathing.

3 Imagine you are holding two golden eggs in your armpits to facilitate relaxation throughout your posture. Maintain a slight curve in every joint to allow your chi to sink.

4 Make sure your buttocks are not protruding or contracted, but held naturally so that your tailbone is in alignment with the rest of your spine.

5 The waist must be loose and relaxed as it links the upper and lower body so they move in coordination.

6 When moving forwards or backwards, make sure your knees never extend over your toes. Never do a posture or movement that is uncomfortable or pushes your body beyond 70 per cent effort.

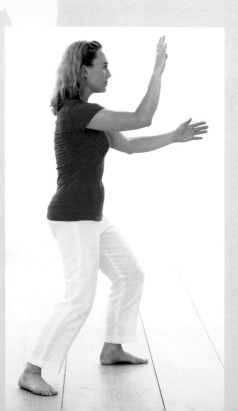

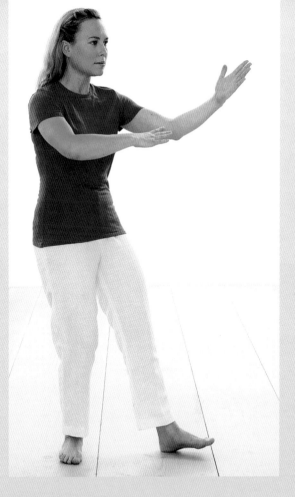

correction of the breath

Breath is one of the most important aspects of chi exercise as through it you gather, direct and circulate your chi. Most people do not breathe deeply enough. The following reminders will help you improve your breathing when practising Chi Kung or T'ai Chi.

1 Always breathe through your nose into your lower abdomen, then let your upper chest expand naturally. On exhalation empty your abdomen and chest simultaneously.

2 To become more conscious of your breath, practise breathing in through your nose and holding your breath for several seconds, then exhaling through your nose. Over time you will become aware of the sensations of chi filling your lungs and circulating throughout your body.

3 Coordinate your breath with your movements when practising Chi Kung and T'ai Chi.

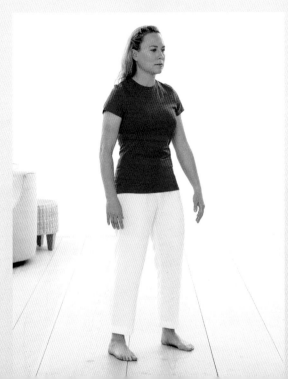

correction of the mind

Without clear intention, it is hard to accomplish anything in life. Your mind will wander and your chi will be unfocused and scattered. When practising chi exercises, have the intention to gather, circulate and balance your chi energy in order to enhance your health and well-being. When practising, keep the following in your consciousness:

1 Practise with a quiet mind and calm spirit.

2 Use your mind to direct the movements of your body and your chi.

3 Stay focused on what you are doing. Pay attention to your breath, posture and movements, and the sensations in your body.

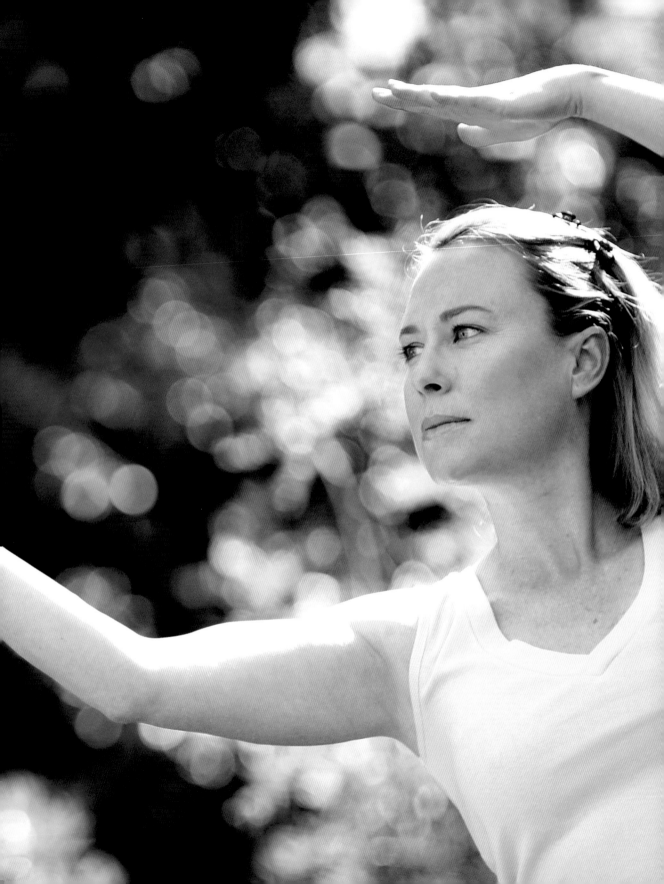

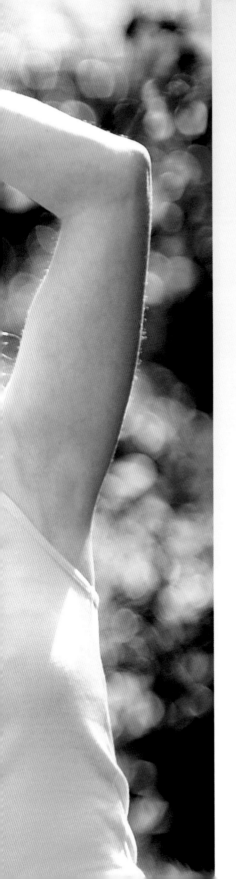

BASIC T'AI CHI AND CHI KUNG EXERCISES

Chi Kung and T'ai Chi are excellent practices for balancing chi energy. If possible, find a quiet place outdoors to practise the following exercises. An ideal location would be a pine forest because conifers have a remarkably calming chi energy. Otherwise, any place with plants, grass and trees would be beneficial. Avoid practising outdoors in stormy weather or when it is excessively hot, or during solar and lunar eclipses, as it is easier to absorb chi from nature when it is in a calm and balanced state.

The Chi Kung exercises can be practised individually, while the T'ai Chi movements should be practised in sequence as they are part of the opening movements of the Simplified Yang Style Form. You can practise Chi Kung or T'ai Chi at any time of day or night, but avoid exercising after a full meal. At that time you need your chi for digestion and you do not want to lead it away from your centre to your extremities.

Wu Chi

This is the fundamental posture – most Chi Kung sequences begin and end with Wu Chi. It honours the full power and primal chi energy of the human being and of the universe. The stance helps to bring you into physical alignment and connect to the source of chi in heaven and earth.

With consistent practice, this exercise will help clear accumulated chronic tension and underlying chi imbalances from your body. As you become more open to the chi energy in the natural environment and your sensitivity to your own chi energy deepens, this practice will take on a joyful quality. You will begin to experience directly the power of the earth below and the vast cosmos above.

1 Begin by standing with your feet shoulder-width apart. Let your head rest lightly on your neck, as if suspended by a thread from above. Relax your eyes and focus ahead but slightly downwards.

2 Lower your chin slightly and relax your jaw, neck, and shoulders. Imagine warm water pouring down from above, dissolving your tension and stiffness.

3 Let your arms curve gently away from your body as if you are holding two golden eggs under your arms. Relax your hands and fingers. Let them hang loosely by your sides. Breathe naturally through your nose into your lower abdomen. As you relax let your breathing deepen.

4 Let your knees relax and sink slightly as if you were about to sit. Feel your feet holding up the full weight of your body. Stand in this position for as long as you are comfortable. Try to build up to 20 minutes a day.

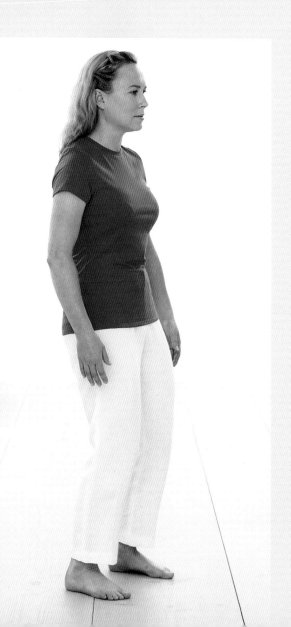

opening the gate of life

This exercise takes its name from a meridian point in the middle of the lower back. Stimulating this important point encourages chi throughout your entire body and releases tension in your hips and torso. It stimulates and balances your kidneys and benefits your lumbar spine. The twisting action of this exercise also massages your internal organs.

1 Start in Wu Chi with your feet shoulder-width apart and knees slightly bent. Let your arms hang naturally at your sides.

2 Twist your hips to the left while shifting your weight to your left foot and raising your right heel. Twist fast enough and with enough energy so that your arms swing on their own with the movement. If you twist with enough force, your right hand will swing up across your chest and slap your left shoulder. Your left hand will swing behind you so that the back of your hand knocks against the centre of your lower back.

3 Now twist your hips to the right, duplicating the complete movement on the opposite side. Start slowly and build up to a continuous motion from side-to-side until you develop a loose, rhythmic swing. The back of each hand will knock against the centre of your lower back. When you have established a rhythm, bend your knees a little and add some bounce as you synchronize with your movement. Do 10 complete swings on each side.

1   2   3

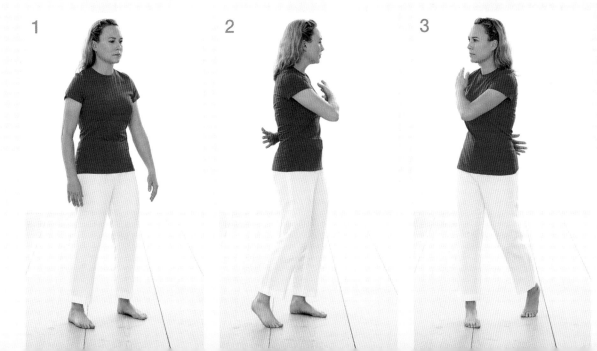

opening and expanding the chest

Practise this exercise to balance your lung and heart chi. It can help with asthma, heart disease, heart palpitations, breathing problems and feelings of pressure in your chest from anxiety and emotional stress. If you have been holding tension in your chest area, and walking around with hunched shoulders, this excellent exercise will relax your body, mind and spirit.

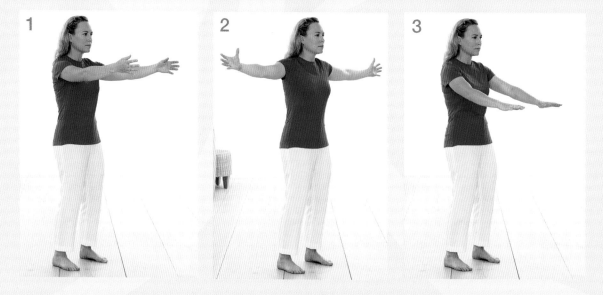

Throughout this exercise, focus on releasing tension in your chest. As you open your arms out to the sides, imagine your heart relaxing and opening. As you inhale, fill your lungs with fresh air. When you exhale, visualize any physical or emotional problems leaving your body as grey smoke. After practising this exercise six times, notice any sensations of energy flow in your heart and lung meridians along the interior of your arms.

1 Stand in the Wu Chi position (see page 102). As you inhale, slowly lift your hands in front of you to shoulder-height, arms outstretched with palms facing one another. Keep your elbows straight, but not locked and let the movement originate from your shoulders, keeping them down and relaxed.

2 Open your arms straight out to the side while you raise your body to full height. Keep your eyes straight ahead and your knees relaxed. Do not squeeze your shoulders together but imagine your arms are lengthening out to the sides.

3 Exhale and close your arms until they are parallel once more. Turn your palms down and let your arms and hands sink back down to your sides as you lower your stance to the starting position. Repeat six times.

moving the rainbow

This gentle exercise will stimulate chi flow along the meridians in your back. It will help relieve lower back pain and help correct poor posture in your upper back and shoulders by gently stretching your muscles. As you practise, imagine that you are moving a beautiful rainbow from side-to-side. Generate a feeling of inner peace and contentment. Allow your worries to dissolve.

1 Stand in the Wu Chi position (see page 102). Inhale and slowly lift your arms in front of you to chest-height parallel to the floor.

2 Move your left arm out to your left side, palm up and lift your right arm above your head with the palm of your hand slightly curving in. At the same time, shift your weight on to your right leg keeping your left foot stationary on the ground, heel raised.

3 Exhale and gradually shift your weight to your left leg, simultaneously raising your left arm above your head with the palm of your hand curving in slightly. Halfway

through the shift, your hands should both be over-head and your whole body should be symmetrical.

4 As you shift your weight to your left leg, let your right hand sink and extend out from your right side, and lift and curve your left arm over your head so that your palm faces the top of your head. The shift from side to side should be flowing and harmonious. Repeat the shift six times to each side. When inhaling, place your weight on your right leg and move your arms to the left; when exhaling place your weight on your left leg and move your arms to the right.

1   2   3   4

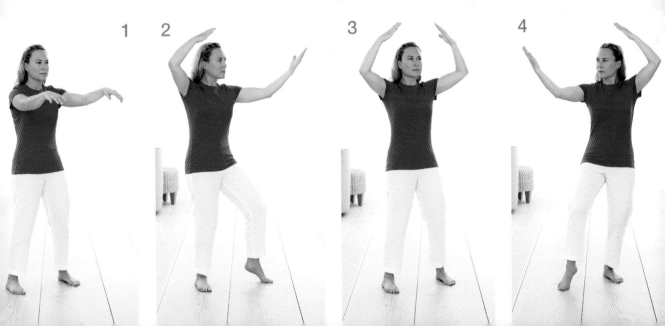

t'ai chi opening posture

As you begin this opening movement of the simplified T'ai Chi form, breathe into your lower abdomen. As you breathe, visualize chi being drawn up from the earth through the bottom and centre of your feet just below the ball. This is the first point on the kidney meridian called Bubbling Well and is the point where yin earth energy enters the body. Visualize your entire body being nourished by earth chi.

1 Stand with feet together, toes slightly pointing out. Relax your shoulders and tuck in the base of your spine. Imagine your head is suspended by a thread. Sink your weight into your right foot, raise your left foot and place it down about shoulder-width from your right foot into Wu Chi position (see page 102).

2 Inhale, and while keeping your arms, wrists and fingers relaxed, allow your arms to float upwards to about chest height. Your forearms should be parallel to the ground and your shoulders relaxed and still.

3 As you breathe out, slowly raise and straighten your fingers. Let your wrists drop so your palms are slightly facing outwards.

4 Now press your palms down until they are hip-height. Let your knees bend slightly and let your weight sink. Your weight should be evenly distributed on both feet.

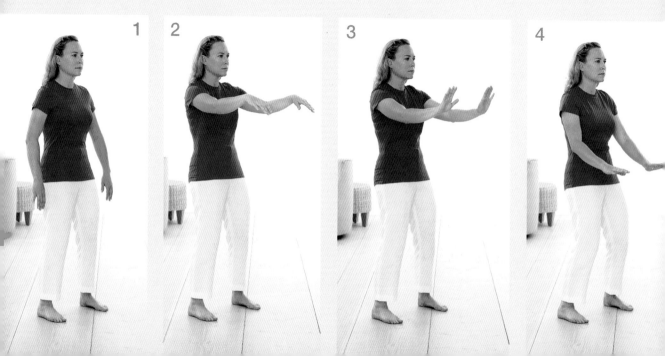

wild horse waves its mane

This is the first movement of the form where you shift your weight to one leg. From here on until the final movement of the form, you would always have your weight on one leg or the other, not both. You begin by placing your arms as if holding on to a ball of chi. The name of this movement suggests that the energy of a wild horse could be at your disposal, if you learn to preserve, manage and balance your chi through diet, exercise and meditation. The wild horse is waving its mane, urging you to take the challenge.

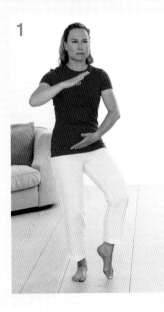 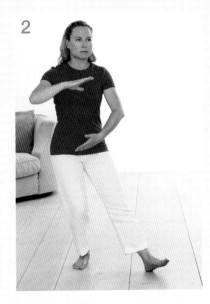 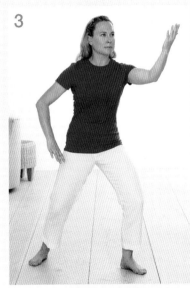

1 Stand in Wu Chi position (see page 102). Turn slightly to your right and shift your weight to your right foot, and bring your left foot close to your right with toes on the ground. Raise your right hand, palm down, to shoulder height, and move your left hand, palm facing up, under your hand as if you were holding a 'ball of chi'.

2 Turn your upper body to your left. Step to the left with your left foot, heel first.

3 Next, shift your weight on to your left leg. You should now be in a forwards lunge position with the left knee bent and your right leg straight. As you shift your weight your hands move apart. Your left hand moves left and up to eye level, palm facing upwards and your right hand falls down to hip level, palm facing down. Your eyes are focused on your left palm.

white crane spreads its wings

This movement signifies grace, beauty and longevity. It represents the search for the Tao in everyday life and the Taoist emphasis on observing and learning from nature. Inspired by early Chi Kung practices based on the movement of birds and animals, White Crane Spreads Its Wings is one of the most beautiful movements in the simplified yang form. The chi moves up from the earth through your left leg and down from the heavens through your upraised right arm or 'wing'.

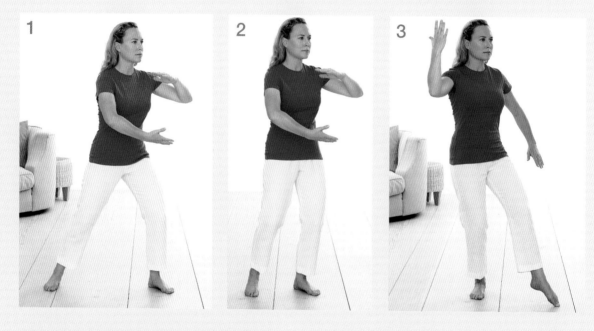

1 From step 3 of Wild Horse Waves Its Mane (see page 107), turn your upper body slightly to the left and bring your left hand down in front of your chest. Turn your right hand over, palm up, bringing it to waist level so that both arms are in 'holding ball of chi position'.

2 Let your right foot take a half-step forwards, then draw your upper body back to shift your weight on to your right leg.

3 Bring your left leg a little forwards with only your toes touching the ground. Your left leg carries no weight. As you shift your weight back, raise your right hand in front of you to the right side of your head, palm facing inwards, and lower your left hand to your left side, palm down. Your eyes are facing forwards.

brush knee and twist step

If you practise T'ai Chi as a martial art, in this movement you would be advancing on your opponent, blocking and brushing aside his or her attack. In a non-martial sense, visualize that you are moving ahead in your life and brushing aside and removing those habits that are compromising your health and chi energy.

1 From step 3 of White Crane Spreads Its Wings (see page 108), turn your upper body to the right, at the same time, sweep your right hand down then up in a curve to ear level, palm facing in. Simultaneously, bring your left hand up in a curve to the right side of your chest, palm facing down, eyes looking at your right hand.

2 Turn your upper body left, take a step forwards with your left foot into a forward lunge. Bring your right hand from behind and push it forwards, level with your right ear, palm facing outward. Let your left hand go down and brush past your left knee to rest beside your left hip, eyes looking forward at the back of your right hand.

3 Bend your right leg and shift your weight backwards on to it, move your upper body back at the same time. Raise the toes of your left foot and turn them slightly out to the left before placing them flat on the floor. Turn your palms inwards, so that you are holding the 'ball of chi'.

4 Bend your left leg, turn your body to the left and shift your weight on to your left foot. Bring your right foot next to your left foot and rest it on its toes. Move your left hand, palm up, to shoulder height while your right hand curves in to chest height, palm down, eyes looking at your left hand. Now repeat steps 2 to 4 on the other side, starting by stepping out with your right foot into a forward lunge.

1 2 3 4

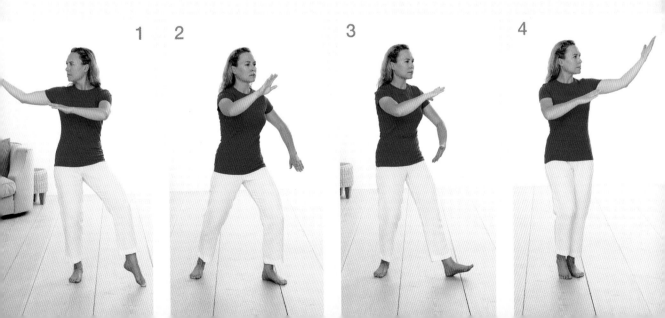

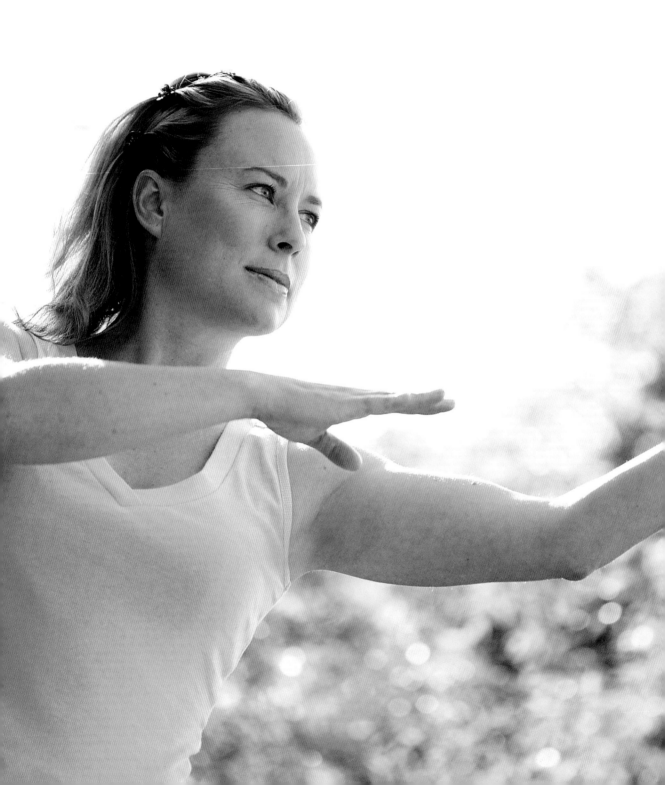

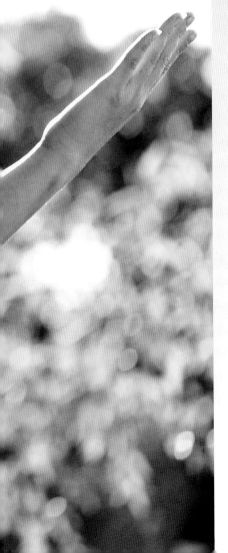

CHI AND SPIRITUAL PRACTICE

In this chapter we will explore the relationship of chi to spiritual practice. We pull together the threads from the previous chapters and see where they fall on the path of the Tao. You will begin to understand how massaging your meridians, eating to enhance your health and practising T'ai Chi or Chi Kung might be related to achieving enlightenment. You will learn to engage the power of your mind in the process of circulating and enhancing chi through various meditation practices. Through meditation, you will bring working with chi to a higher level and bring your self closer to nature, the universe and the experience of Tao.

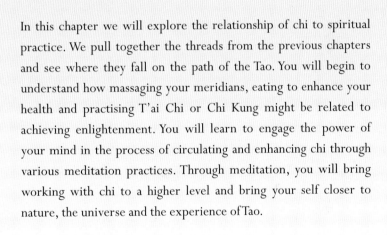

chi and the path of Tao

For thousands of years, Taoists have explored the meaning and nature of the universe. They observed that the universe is not a thing but a process of constant change in which everything is interconnected. They called this process the One or the Tao. The One signifies the state of non-differentiation of the universe, the primordial state of great unity.

key concept

The Taoist spiritual path includes many of the chi health practices covered in this book.

As the word Taoism suggests, following the path of the Tao or the Great Unity is a key concept within this religion. The Taoist Path is sometimes referred to as Keeping the One or Guarding the One, which is defined as a three-step process. Health, longevity and spiritual growth are achieved by first emulating nature and eliminating imbalances within oneself. Then, self-purified and made healthy and whole, one enters into a renewed relationship with the environment. After intensive spiritual exploration and practice, one becomes merged with the One or the Tao.

The following is a short explanation of the Path of Guarding the One that will show where the practices you have been learning fall on the Taoist path to realization of the One.

Stage 1: Guarding the One

In the first stage, you work on becoming whole by finding the One within yourself. You work diligently to eliminate the imbalances and energy blockages within your body and mind. Once you have reached a place of wholeness, you can interact more freely with the world around you and also explore the nature of cosmos. The practices in this book relating to achieving health and longevity through working with chi, are practices for stage one of the Taoist Path. Through Chi Kung, T'ai Chi, meridian massage and diet, you begin to bring your body into balance and wholeness. You work to synchronize your mind, body and breath. Your goal is to achieve optimum health and chi flow throughout your body, and absolute peacefulness and purity of mind.

Stage 2: Chaos

To enter the next stage, you leave behind all the chi-enhancing practices you have learned and enter a state of chaos. From the healthy state you have achieved, you abandon yourself into experiencing the world. Playing music serves as an example of how you might do this. When you learn to play an instrument, you become proficient by practising the notes and scales. You then memorize a piece of music, which allows you to play within the prescribed pattern of notes. But if you want to truly understand a piece of music you transcend the notes and simply enter into the music. This abandonment is the desired chaos, the state that Taoists achieve by first mastering the preliminary purifying practices, and then forgetting them for a more profound state of being.

The elimination of imbalances in your body through massage, diet and exercise prepares you for higher spiritual realization of the One or the Tao.

Stage 3: The Return

You no longer react to whatever happens around you; instead, you become one with it. If you are driving a car on familiar roads, you may become so lost in thought that you may not even be aware of the drive until you arrive home. At this point the distinction between your route and the act of driving disappears. You become the car and the road and everything along the way. Likewise, in this third stage, the distinction between the Tao and the experience disappears. At this stage, you have finally returned to the state of complete stillness in which you are one with the Tao.

Taoist meditation on guarding the one

When you realize that everything in life is an expression of the One Unity you can relax. You can feel safe in the world. Good news, bad news – it is all part of the same thing. Everything is an expression of the One. When you are able to relax into the Tao your chi flows smoothly and your body and mind are in harmony. Even if you have not actually experienced the One, knowing it is possible to do so brings a sense of peace.

Meditation is one of the best practices for the health of your body and mind.

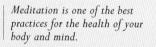

early meditations

Instructions for a meditation on the first phase of the path Guarding the One are found in one of the earliest Taoist classics on inner cultivation, called Neije or Inward Training, which dates from around 500 BCE. First it directs you to expand your heart-mind and release it. Then you are asked to relax your chi and allow it to extend. Finally, when your body is calm and unmoving, you are advised to discard any of the myriad disturbances that pull you from a realization of the One.

This method for spiritual growth is as relevant today as it was 3,000 years ago – you are asked to decrease worldly distractions and the tendency to look outside yourself for answers. You are advised to focus inwards and cultivate clarity and stillness. In this way, you may have a chance to become one with the One or the Tao.

guarding the one meditation

Guarding the One is often preceded by preliminary practices to encourage chi flow. Before beginning this meditation, it is helpful to massage your meridians until you feel the glow of chi flowing throughout your body.

1 Sit comfortably, either cross-legged on a mat or with your back straight in a chair. Place your hands on your lower abdomen. Place your tongue against your upper palette behind your teeth and lower your eyes, leaving them slightly open.

2 Bring your attention inwards to the centre of your head, to seal off any input from your senses. Take long, deep, rhythmic breaths through your nose and bring your focus to the relaxed rising and falling of your lower abdomen.

3 Have the intention to remain in deep absorption and be receptive to the mysteriousness and ineffability of the One.

4 Do not be discouraged if thoughts intervene; just keep returning your attention to the stillness within. With time and many meditation sessions, the distracting thoughts and sensations will diminish and you will reach a state of clarity and stillness. From that clarity and stillness, you will discover inner realms that only your own experience will fully reveal.

5 With practice, you may eventually come to the experience of emptiness. And from the experience of emptiness, you have a chance to attain the state of realizing the One or the Tao.

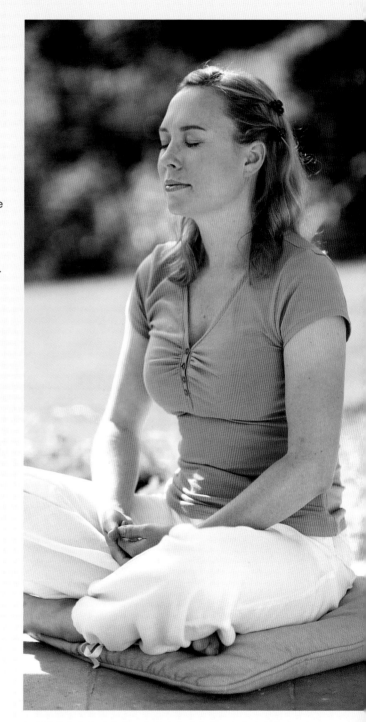

the inner smile

The Inner Smile, a secret of inner Taoist soul alchemy, is a self-healing meditation that utilizes your heart and the energy of love to communicate with your internal organs and pathways, dissolve chi blockages and facilitate chi circulation. An authentic smile transmits loving energy and has the power to heal. It magically opens your chi flow.

inner smile meditation

Since this is a long meditation, it is best to record the steps ahead of time and play it back for yourself when you are ready to practise the Inner Smile.

1 Stand in Wu Chi stance (see page 102) or sit comfortably on the edge of a chair with your feet flat on the floor. Keep your spine straight yet relaxed.

2 Relax your forehead and become aware of your third eye, the midpoint between your eyebrows. Imagine being in a beautiful place where someone you love is smiling lovingly at you. Take in the warmth of that person's smile and respond with a smile of your own. Feel your eyes smiling and relaxing.

3 Draw this warm smiling energy into your third eye and allow it to open. As it accumulates, your smiling energy will eventually overflow into your body.

4 Allow the smiling energy to flow down from your third eye through your face and down through your neck to your thymus gland and heart. Spend as much time here as you need to feel your heart and thymus relax and expand as you shower it with your loving energy.

5 Next, radiate your smile to your solid organs – your lungs, liver, pancreas, spleen, kidneys, sexual organs and reproductive system. Spend time smiling at each one and let each one know how much they are loved and appreciated.

6 Bring your awareness back to yourself and recharge your smile by drawing more loving chi energy into your third eye. Swish your tongue around your mouth to create saliva. Swallow in three gulps. With your inner smile, follow the saliva down your oesophagus through your stomach and gall bladder. Relax your smiling energy into your small intestine, large intestine and rectum.

7 Recharge your smile through your third eye. Then, smile into both hemispheres of your brain, your pituitary, thalamus and pineal glands. Smile down the inside your spinal column, descending one vertebra at a time, smiling on to each until you have reached the coccyx.

8 Return to your eyes again. Smile down your whole body and shower it with your loving energy. Feel your body responding and appreciating your love. Try to maintain this feeling as you go about your day.

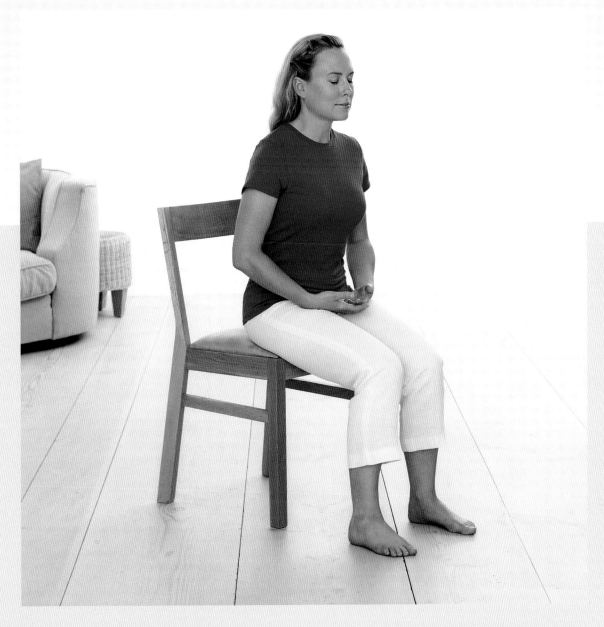

9 Now collect your smiling energy at your navel, about 4 cm (1½ inches) inside your body. Mentally move that energy in an outward spiral 36 times without going above the diaphragm or beneath the pubic bone. Women spiral counter-clockwise, men clockwise.

Next, reverse the direction and bring it back into the navel, circling it 24 times. The energy is now safely stored in your navel, available to you whenever you need it and for whatever part of your body needs it. You have now completed the Inner Smile.

the microcosmic orbit

This meditation is an ancient Taoist chi meditation that is said to connect you to heaven chi, Cosmic chi, (the chi of your Higher Self) and Earth chi, adding more chi to your Three Treasures – your physical, energy and spirit bodies.

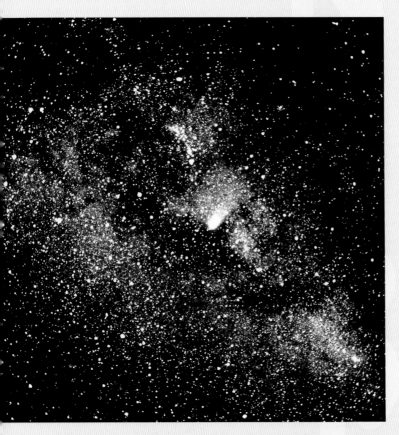

This Taoist meditation practice works by opening the Microcosmic Orbit, which follows the path created by two additional meridians in the body that run up the centre of the back and down the centre of the front of the body. The front channel is called the Conception Vessel, the back channel called the Governor Vessel. They join to form a circuit of continuous energy flow called the Microcosmic Orbit. It is said that the circulation of chi in the Microcosmic Orbit is the first chi circulation that occurs in our body as we develop in our mother's womb. The Microcosmic Orbit is the main energetic circuit of the body and feeds all the other channels.

The Microcosmic Orbit meditation connects your chi to that of the entire universe.

microcosmic orbit meditation

The Microcosmic Orbit meditation is a wonderful Taoist practice for integrating your body and mind. In this meditation you will learn that where the mind moves, chi will follow.

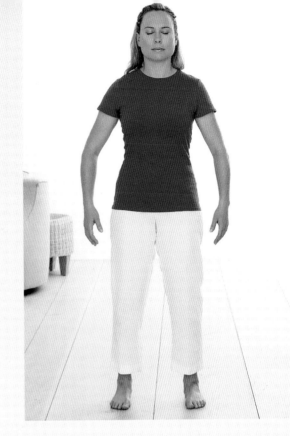

1 Stand in Wu Chi stance (see page 102) or sit on the edge of a chair with your feet flat on the floor. Clasp your hands together and rest them on your lap. Close your eyes, calm your mind and regulate your breath. Focus your attention on your abdomen and breathe into it. Imagine warmth and chi energy filling your lower abdomen in the form of a golden light. With each breath imagine your reservoir of chi growing.

When you feel your lower abdomen is filled with chi begin to move the chi or golden light with your mind to your navel area.

2 When you feel it has arrived at that point, move the golden light with your mind to your sexual centre, or the Sperm/Ovary Palace.

3 When the feeling is stable and the energy there is full, use your mind to guide energy down to the perineum or Gate of Life and Death.

4 Visualize the golden light and energy gradually passing through your coccyx. When you feel the energy has moved through this pass, visualize it rising up to where your ribs meet with your spine, known as the Door of Life.

5 When the energy has filled this point, move it up to your lower mid back, to your adrenal centre, where your adrenal glands sit atop your kidneys. When you are ready, move on up to the Jade Pillow at the base of your brain, through your crown and down to your third eye between your eyebrows.

6 Connect the Conception Vessel and the Governor Vessel by bringing your attention to the tip of your tongue. Touch the tip of your tongue to your palate connecting the two channels. Press and release your tongue against your palate 36 times. This activates the palate point.

7 Let the golden energy sink down through your palate and tongue into your throat centre, before moving down to your heart.

8 From your heart, draw the energy down through your Middle Elixir Field in the solar plexus, and complete the Orbit back at your navel. Continue to circulate your chi through the Microcosmic Orbit in this way at least nine times.

9 The Microcosmic Orbit opens up, energizes and distributes your natural energy throughout the body. When you are finished visualize collecting the chi energy and storing it in your navel area.

essence of heaven

Taoists appreciated nature and preferred to be in its quiet presence away from the distractions of everyday living. This was conducive to accessing the chi of sunshine, water, trees and plants, and learning from and aligning with the rhythms and cycles of natures.

essence of heaven meditation

The Essence of Heaven meditation is focused on the yang energy of the sun. This meditation is practised outdoors in the sunshine, preferably around trees and plants. Ancient Taoist sages believed that the yang Essence from Heaven chi is transferred from the sun's rays to the body. Modern scientists, who may know nothing about chi, have concurred that it is important to be in the presence of sunlight for at least 20 minutes a day. The sun's rays make chemical changes in the body, producing Vitamin D essential for calcium absorption, and activate the production of hormones important for sleep.

1 Stand outside in the early hours of the morning before sunrise when the air is fresher and cleaner, and face east. If possible, find a spot where you can stand directly on the earth.

2 Standing with feet shoulder-width apart, let your head rest lightly on your neck. Relax your eyes and focus them ahead at the horizon. Lower your chin slightly and relax your jaw, neck and shoulders.

3 Scan your body and dissolve any tension and stiffness. Let your arms curve gently away from your body as if you were holding two golden eggs under your arms. Relax your hands and fingers. Let them hang loosely downwards.

4 Breathe naturally through your nose into your lower abdomen. As you relax let your breathing deepen.

5 Let your knees relax and sink slightly as if you were about to sit. Feel your feet holding up the full weight of your body and connecting with earth chi.

6 When the sun appears on the horizon, place the palms of your hands against your abdomen, lean slightly forwards from the waist and breathe out through your nose to empty your lungs of stale air.

7 Inhale fresh air combined with the yang essence of the rising sun through your nostrils directing your mind and breath to your abdomen. Visualize the sun's purifying chi energy entering your body through your nose. Exhale the stale, impure air. Exhale and inhale in this way for three complete breaths.

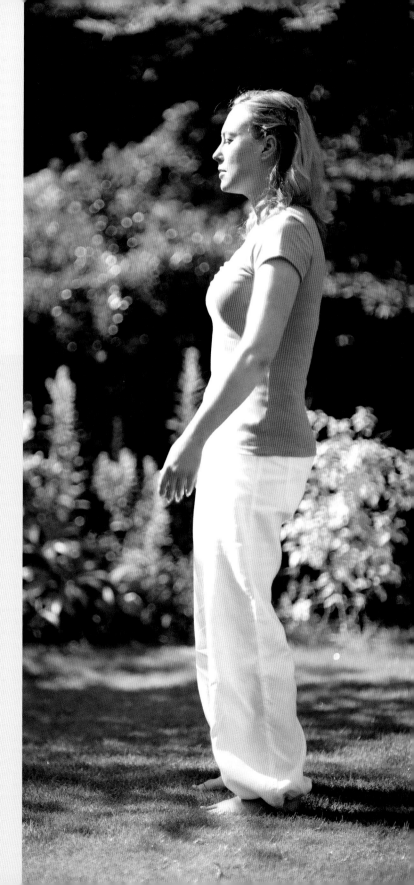

8 Inhale the chi of the sun deep into
   your abdomen for a slow count of five,
   hold your breath for another count of
   five and then exhale slowly at the
   same speed. Breath into your
   abdomen in this way, storing the
   sun's chi energy, until your abdomen
   begins to feel warm.

9 At noon return to the same spot and
   face south (north in the southern
   hemisphere). Inhale deeply into your
   abdomen and this time swallow the air
   you breathe in. Exhale any impurities.

10 In the evening, face the setting sun
   and swallow the air your breathe in,
   and when the sun sets, take in the
   last traces of the sun's chi energy by
   breathing in and swallowing.

three fields of elixir

This meditation is based on the three centres in the body or Tan Tiens, which translates as Fields of Elixir. The fields are areas in your body where your chi has accumulated and is stored in a reservoir. The Three Treasures – jing (essence), chi (energy) and shen (spirit) are centred in and operate from the Three Elixir Fields. Your Three Treasures also represent three forms of your chi – body, mind and spirit chi.

upper field of elixir

The upper Field of Elixir is located in the middle of the brain, just below where the soft spot of your head was when you were born, and behind the area between your eyes called the third eye. This is the Tan Tien of your shen or spirit, one of the Three Treasures of the Human Being. The spirit is associated with heavenly chi. It is yang, expansive, having to do with the vastness of the cosmos, the stars, planets and universe. It is spiritual, transcendent and boundless, and in some ways incomprehensible.

middle field of elixir

The middle Tan Tien is located in the middle of the chest at the solar plexus. It is sometimes called the heart Tan Tien and is the residence of the heart-mind. This is the place of thought, memory and emotions, a place of heart and mind combined. This is the place of the integration of thinking and feeling. It is the home of your third Treasure, chi.

lower field of elixir

The lower Field of Elixir is most often simply called the Tan Tien and is located about 5 cm (2 inches) below the navel. It is associated with jing, or essence. It is yin, having to do with the body, the earth, density, contraction, DNA and sexuality. It is quiet and dark and has to do with the earth itself – rocks, sand, lakes, weather.

The Taoist world view associates the body with earth and the feminine, the spirit with heaven and the masculine. Chi, the life-force, the breath of life is said to be the child born from the merging of the two. Between heaven and earth all living things emerge.

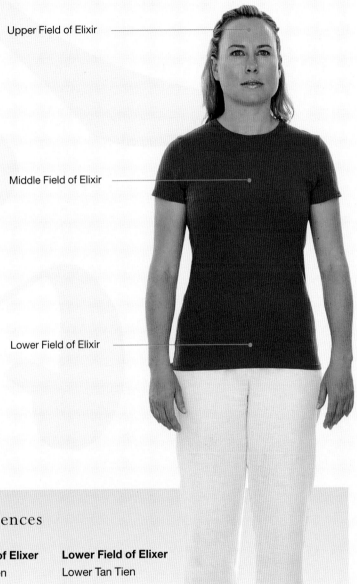

Upper Field of Elixir

Middle Field of Elixir

Lower Field of Elixir

fields of elixir correspondences

Upper Field of Elixer	Middle Field of Elixer	Lower Field of Elixer
Upper Tan Tien	Middle Tan Tien	Lower Tan Tien
Shen	Chi	Jing
Spirit	Heart-mind	Body
Heaven	Life	Earth
Yang	Harmony	Yin

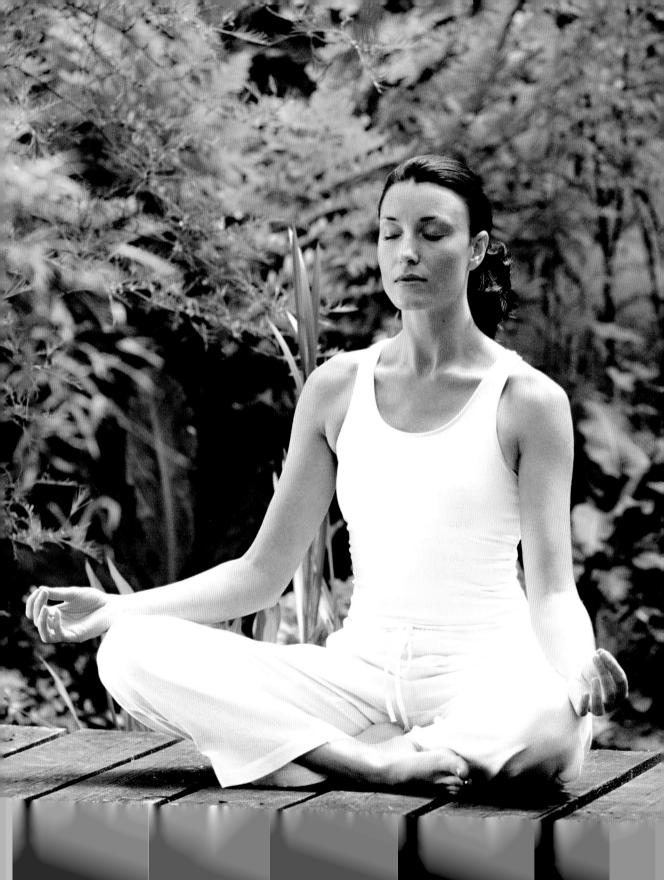

three fields of elixir meditation

1 Record this meditation and play it back when you are ready to meditate. Sit in meditation posture, either on a cushion or on the edge of a chair. If possible meditate outdoors near water and trees. Have your spine straight and shoulders relaxed. Rest your hands comfortably in your lap or on your knees. Scan your body for any tension and release it.

2 Breathe deeply for a few minutes to calm your mind. Draw your awareness into the centre of your mind and close off all external distractions. When your breath and mind are quiet, begin to meditate on the following visualization.

3 Move your focus to your Upper Field of Elixir, in the space behind your third eye. Concentrate on this point. Visualize the point beginning to glow with a white light. Imagine that point as a brilliant crystal with its many facets reflecting the sunlight. Acknowledge this as the Treasure of your spirit, the seat of your creativity and intuition. Breathe into that point. Feel its expansive yang quality and its connection to heaven chi and the mysteries of deep space and the incomprehensible vastness of the cosmos. Concentrate for a moment at this point and imagine your spirit being released.

4 Now bring your awareness to your Lower Field of Elixir, about 5 cm (2 inches) below your navel and 30 per cent of your body-width inwards. Imagine a warm yellow glow emanating from your Lower Tan Tien. This is the home of the Treasure of your jing, your essence that you inherited from your parents and your ancestors before them. It is the home of your body – peaceful, dark and yin. Sperm and egg are produced here. It is the expression of Earth chi, dense, concentrated, substantive. Breathe deeply into your lower Tan Tien and intend that your body be healed of any illness.

5 Feel your yang, heaven Tan Tien, your Upper Field of Elixir and your yin Earth Tan Tien and your Lower Field of Elixir being drawn to each other like poles on a magnet. Move your awareness to your Middle Tan Tien, your Middle Field of Elixir, where they join to give birth to your third Treasure, your body, your chi – the home of your heart-mind. Now focus on clearing your mind and emotions of any stress, worry or judgment. Do not cling to any thoughts that may arise. Allow a sense of peace and harmony to spread from the middle of your chest throughout your entire body. Imagine your thinking and feeling aspects merging and operating as one entity. Allow your heart-mind to lead your body and spirit.

6 Bring your awareness to all three Fields of Elixir simultaneously. Imagine all three glowing with light and warmth. Generate a sense of gratitude and deep appreciation for your Three Treasures and commit to cherishing them for the rest of your life.

index

acknowledgements

Special Photography
©Octopus Publishing Group Limited/Ruth Jenkinson

All other photography
Alamy/Chris Hermann 92; /Mary Evans Picture Library 10; /Mike Abrahams 27; /Pat Behnke 15. **Bridgeman Art Library** 11. **Corbis UK Ltd** 18, /Eric Cahan 31; /Javier Pierini 30; /Mike McQueen 96; /Sergio Pitamitz 26; /Tetra Images 33. **Getty Images**/Barry Yee 35. **Octopus Publishing Group Limited**/Bill Reavell 75; /Frank Adam 67; /Gareth Sambidge 60, 62; /Laura Forrester 61; /Lis Parsons 72; /Marcus Harper 44; /Mike Prior 1, 13 top right, 21, 97, 112, 113, 114; /Peter Pugh-Cook 65; /Russell Sadur 19, 32, 76, 83; /Stephen Conroy 68 top left, 69, 80; /William Lingwood 66, 68 bottom right, 73, 79; /William Reavell 63, 74. **Photolibrary**/Dynamic Graphics (UK) 124. **Royalty-Free Images** 14, 29; /BananaStock 34; /PhotoDisc 28, 64, 78, 93, 118. **Shutterstock**/B.S. Karan 16; /Cora Reed 51; /Jarvis Gray 46; /Jiri Vaclavek 45; /Juriah Mosin 82; /Siloto 43; /Valentin Russanov 42. **Tse Qigong Centre** 22, 94, 95.

Executive Editor Sandra Rigby
Editor Kerenza Swift
Executive Art Editor Sally Bond
Designer Elizabeth Healey
Photographer Ruth Jenkinson
Picture Research Taura Riley
Senior Production Controller
  Simone Nauerth